The 30-Minute Runner

SMART TRAINING FOR BUSY BEGINNERS

DUNCAN LARKIN
Foreword by DR. MIKE MORENO

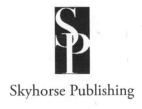

Skyhorse Publishing

Copyright © 2018 by Duncan Larkin
Foreword © 2018 by Dr. Mike Moreno

All rights reserved. No part of this book may be reproduced in any manner without the express written consent of the publisher, except in the case of brief excerpts in critical reviews or articles. All inquiries should be addressed to Skyhorse Publishing, 307 West 36th Street, 11th Floor, New York, NY 10018.

Skyhorse Publishing books may be purchased in bulk at special discounts for sales promotion, corporate gifts, fund-raising, or educational purposes. Special editions can also be created to specifications. For details, contact the Special Sales Department, Skyhorse Publishing, 307 West 36th Street, 11th Floor, New York, NY 10018 or info@skyhorsepublishing.com.

Skyhorse® and Skyhorse Publishing® are registered trademarks of Skyhorse Publishing, Inc.®, a Delaware corporation.

Visit our website at www.skyhorsepublishing.com.

10 9 8 7 6 5 4 3 2 1

Library of Congress Cataloging-in-Publication Data is available on file.

Cover design by Tom Lau
Cover photo credit iStock

ISBN: 978-1-5107-2132-6
Ebook ISBN: 978-1-5107-2133-3

Printed in the United States of America

I'm writing this book to honor every runner who has ever come across the finish line in dead-last place. I've run for over thirty years and have taken part in hundreds of races. While it's wonderful to see the look of exaltation on the winners' faces, especially after a hard-fought sprint to the finish-line tape, it's something else entirely to wait till the very end of the race to see that very last person come across the line. If you've never seen it happen, try it. Pat this person on the back and show your support.

You'll learn a lot about running.

Almost every last-place finisher I've seen has tears streaming down their face. They have worked so hard for that moment. It's not easy for some to come in last, but they never seem to care.

They did it.

They overcame incredible mental and physical obstacles. They resisted the temptation to quit.

They persevered.

This is a book about running for beginners, and so it's appropriate to dedicate it to this brave group of athletes. Those who finish last will always teach me the true meaning of this sport. It's not about winning; it's about simply doing—pushing the boundaries and resisting the temptation to quit.

Their dedication deserves all of our respect.

CONTENTS

FOREWORD

"Change" is such a scary word, no matter to what it refers. When we think about our health—I mean really, really think about our health—it comes down to some very basic principles. Two of those big principles are diet and exercise. But where do I start? How do I get motivated? Who do I lean on when I don't know where to go? So many of these answers are priceless. For all of us the answers are different. But I can say one thing, what Duncan Larkin has done in terms of introducing people to change as it applies to exercise is remarkable.

I've been a practicing family medicine physician for twenty years. I've had the fortune of being heavily involved in the weight-loss and wellness industry. I love what I do. I struggle every day, not only with my patients but also with myself. Nothing is easy. When I think about changing habits, whether it's smoking cessation or starting a new exercise program or diet or maybe something simple like starting to drink more water and be more hydrated, I realize these tasks can be very challenging. Duncan has outlined and produced a very reasonable and doable program to help you get back on track. Whether you were a high-end athlete and you're trying to get back into shape or just trying to get started with any exercise program, this book is for you.

I've known Duncan for several years, and I respect his work and his passion. We have collaborated and shared ideas over the years in terms of getting healthy. His dedication to the cause is amazing. Believe me, no one has an easy go of it. It's amazing how being healthy really encompasses some very basic principles. Trying to get started or trying to maintain good habits is a daily challenge.

One of the things I hear from my patients every day is, "I'm getting old," to which I reply, "We all are, and the day you aren't getting older is the day you really have a problem." Honestly, the health of this country has really gone south in the past several years. We all need to lean on each other—on our friends, family members, loved one, even strangers. I hope reading this book can get you going towards a new you. Baby steps is such an under-statement. Believe me, the concept of basic baby steps is the way to succeed when trying to make any changes in your life. Enjoy Duncan's approach. He may be just the answer you need—maybe the answer we all need—to get started down that scary pathway to better health.

—Dr. Mike Moreno, author of *The 17 Day Diet*

Chapter 1

COMMIT

Congratulations on taking the first step towards wellness. For one reason or another, you've put this book into your hands. Why? *Because you seek change.* Something is missing in your life. You want to improve your inner and outer beauty. You want to be well. You want to feel better about yourself. You don't want to just exist; you want to *thrive*.

You know that life can be about so much more if you're physically and mentally healthier. If you can run (or walk) 30 minutes a day, that day will *mean* something. You'll have accomplished something. You'll gain confidence. And after you put in more miles, you'll lose weight and begin to eat healthier. Life will be more fulfilling than it was.

So here you are on the verge of making a lasting change to your life. It's not easy to take that first step. It's far easier to keep those resolutions in your head—to say to yourself that you'll commit to losing weight and embracing a healthier way of life next week or next month—*some other time,* but not today. You see runners out on the roads and you've imagined yourself as one, *but not today.* Today is about everything else going on in your busy life, and tomorrow is that time when things will magically turn around, right?

But here you are. You've actually done something to turn those good thoughts into action; you've gone and found a book—the right book—to spur you to action.

Congratulations!

It may not seem like much. You aren't sweating or sore from reading a few sentences; you aren't gutting through the last mile of your first training run, but trust me, what you are doing now is just as important, so don't stop. Go, go, go—full speed ahead. Read on. Do what you've been unable to do thus far: commit to making a healthy change.

First things first: this is a book for all types of beginners. I didn't write it just for the clinically obese or for those who've never donned a pair of running shoes. It simply is a book for busy people who want to learn how to run. It can also be for those who used to run and need to get back into shape. It's a book that justifies and explains all the wondrous things that 30 minutes of daily running, or walking if need be, can do for your mind and body and how you can make the best of this magic half hour. It's not your typical how-to running book, though, which means I'm not going to overwhelm you with pages and pages of physiology behind the sport and a bunch of complicated training schedules that leave you scratching your head. I want this book to be a quick read but also something that stays close by for those difficult moments when you need motivation and education—when the proverbial wind is out of your sails.

I've structured this book into six chapters based on the key elements required of you to transform into a happy and healthy 30-minute-a-day runner. You'll notice that these elements are all action verbs that runners need to have in their daily lexicon: commit, learn, train, conquer, sustain, and thrive. After you've read the last page, you should have a basic understanding of what running is, how your body reacts to the stresses and strains of running (**Learn**), what you need to do daily to improve your running (**Train**), how to power through when motivation is flagging (**Conquer**), what you need to do to make it across the finish line in your first 5K race (**Sustain**), and how to make running a part of your life for the rest of your life (**Thrive**). This book will equip you with all the basics you need to build up from zero minutes to 30 minutes for three days or more a week.

So let's start with the book's first principle: **Commit**. You already have this book in your hands and I've already congratulated you for turning the first few pages, but now it's time to do something you probably didn't expect in a running book: I'm going to make you sign a contract. The deal you are about to make is with yourself. I'm just the person who's drawn up the terms for you. You may be scratching your head and wondering why I'm asking you to sign a contract with yourself. This may seem completely crazy, but if you've ever embarked on something big— whether it be getting married or buying a house—you've got to eventually stare at a piece of paper that requires a deep breath, some careful consideration, and a confident signature. A formal contract provides that all-important structure to ensure that you hold up your end of the bargain. In this case, you're going to hold up your end of the bargain while battling against the forces of self-doubt, excuses, and just plain laziness, which are the three culprits that get in the way of our wellness. This important commitment is going to be between your mind and your body. Both the mind and the body have to work together in order to succeed as a runner. And there will inevitably be a time when one or both will want out of the deal. That's why you've got this contract. It specifically includes the following elements and conditions:

- **Perseverance:** By signing this contract, you will commit to enduring through struggle and strife. The mind will come up with a million reasons and excuses why 30 minutes of daily running or walking isn't a priority. Out on the roads, it will try to talk you into quitting, but you have to persevere. You have to realize that you can make it—and you will.

- **Passion:** Your name on the dotted line means that you are making a *total* commitment to living a healthier life. And a total commitment can't happen without passion. Recognize that the moment you take to the roads or trails for your first run you are forever a runner, and no one can take that away from you. From that point forward, you commit to embrace the sport for everything that it is and you learn as much as you can about it. You seek improvement with a smile on your face and will never forget that the darkness that is pain and suffering is ended with the dawning of progress.

- **Patience:** The body doesn't change overnight. The results of your hard work will pay off at some point, but that could be a long time, depending on how you've been taking care of yourself up till now. You have to trust that this change will happen. And with trust must come a mind-set to reject the notion that wellness has nothing to do with instant gratification. You have to slowly put in the time and the work to realize the results.

- **Prioritization:** Running isn't magic. You have to simply get out and do it—nearly every day, working up to 30 minutes—in order to improve. All of us lead incredibly busy lives, and with a busy life comes prioritization. Running and wellness have to be daily priorities just as eating, drinking, and sleeping are. Your signature to this contract indicates you are going to prioritize your running. You won't make excuses; you'll make it happen, because you believe in yourself.

Once you have signed the contract (see page 6), I want you to cut it out of this book and post it up somewhere prominent—a place that you will see every day so that you can remind yourself of the important journey you're on. Perhaps tape it up on your bathroom mirror so that you can see it every day. Or go buy a frame for it and hang it on your wall. Make this document something you're proud of. Show it to your friends and loved ones. Brag about it, because the day that you complete your first 5K with your head held high will be the day that all that work will have been for something good and decent.

30-Minute Daily Running Contract

I, _____, hereby attest that on _____ I signed a contract with myself to run or walk at least 30 minutes a day for as many days of the week as I can. My signature on this document attests to my perseverance, passion, patience, and prioritization to improve my health and make a commitment to wellness. On _____ I am planning to run my first 5K. I am aiming to run it in _____.

Signed,

_____

Shifting Your Equilibrium

With your contract in hand, you should now know something about what it means to make such an important change in your life like this. Any lifestyle change, from quitting smoking to a New Year's resolution like committing to shed a few pounds, requires what I call "shifting the equilibrium." Webster's dictionary defines equilibrium as "a state of balance between opposing forces." If you haven't run before, think of this state as where you are now. Imagine your physical equilibrium as your daily routine that's comprised of three key components—what and how much you eat, how much and how frequently you exercise, and how much you sleep.

By picking up this book, you most likely aren't satisfied with your weight and your fitness, but yet you have settled into your unique routine. This is your personal equilibrium.

Take a few minutes to think about your current equilibrium by answering the following 10 questions:

1. The number of minutes you exercise every day: _____
2. The number of days a week that you exercise: _____
3. Describe your eating habits: _____
4. What types of food do you eat most often? _____
5. How often do you snack during the day? _____
6. What kind of snacks do you eat? _____
7. How much water do you drink? _____
8. How much sleep do you get per night? _____
9. Estimate how many hours a day that you are sedentary (watching screens or sitting at your desk): _____
10. How many extra pounds would you like to lose thanks to running? _____

For better or worse, what you've just written out is your routine. It's YOU. It's your personal equilibrium. Over time, this routine has most likely led to your current state.

But given the fact that you now have this book in your hands, you probably want to be healthier. You want to run for at least 30 minutes a day. Maybe you want to finish your first 5K. In order to do this, you need to *shift* your equilibrium. Bear in mind that to do this, you are going to have to deal with opposing forces. In other words, becoming a first-time 5K runner means you are going to encounter some serious resistance.

This resistance, or friction, stops most of us in our tracks. It's why we eventually quit diets and resume unhealthy habits a few weeks after January 1.

Friction hurts, so buckle up and get ready.

The only way you can shift your equilibrium is to be disciplined and do the work; the work does not get done by itself. This means making the right choices when you eat, getting to bed early when you'd like to stay up, and showing up on the roads, tracks, or trails to do the workout when you'd much rather be in bed or binge-watching your favorite show in front of your iPad.

At first when you begin this shift, your body will rebel. It is going to feel strange to you. If you've never worked out before, just the idea of lacing up running shoes and heading out for a walk or a run will feel completely alien to you—so will eating healthy foods or getting down on the floor of your living room and doing some cross-training exercises.

Most of us are creatures of habit, so this equilibrium shift isn't going to be easy. You have to be on the lookout for it and prepare yourself—mentally and physically—for the challenges you will face by taking your body out of its routine.

Here are five tips to gird yourself for the great equilibrium shift you are about to encounter.

- **Vocalize the shift with your network.** Tell your friends, family, and coworkers what you are doing. Show them your newly signed contract. Post about it on social media and generate some "likes" about your bold move. The more you communicate what you are doing, the easier it will be to follow up on your commitment when those winds of resistance blow your way. The more friction you encounter during the shift, the more you should lean on your network of support. This network can help you through the difficult periods. Conversely, giving support to them during their own equilibrium shifts can also help you feel better about yours.

- **Make the changes gradual and take things one day at a time.** As you will see in later chapters of this book, I strongly believe in the principles of incrementalism. Small steps are easier to take on this journey than long ones. As you read this book, seek to apply the schedules and principles in bite-sized chunks. Overreaching will only encounter that proportional amount of counterresistance.

- **Remember that your equilibrium shift gets easier with every passing day, as long as you stay disciplined.** Whether you realize it or not, as long as you stay consistent, every day you run, eat healthier, and cross-train means a day that you are successful in making the big shift and your mind and body will begin to accept the new "normal."

- **Embrace the struggle.** Even if you fall short attaining some of your goals, remember that nothing that matters ever comes easy. Positive change requires real work. You will experience suffering, and while you can't control this, you can control your attitude along the way. Be proud of what you are doing. It takes true courage to shift the equilibrium. Others make excuses when they encounter those forces of resistance and eventually give up. But that's not you. Suffering comes with the territory, and you will be better for it. Take on the challenge with a positive attitude.

- **As you improve, you will encounter more equilibrium shifts.** Once you start making healthier choices and exercising regularly, your routine will change for the better. But to continue to improve, you will still have to encounter those pesky forces of resistance. Being mindful of this truism will help as you embark on your journey.

A Personal Story

A lot of how-to running books are written by elite runners and coaches—those at the very top of the sport who can sometimes appear to look down on beginners and dispel wisdom to the unenlightened as if they, the fast ones, have all the answers.

Know that I'm not this kind of runner.

I'm one of you.

When I was in the fifth grade, several of my classmates teased me because of my weight. I was a bit chunky, and the ridicule was almost too much to bear. I struggled and, in middle school, decided to try my hand at wrestling—an individual sport that, for some reason, I thought I'd be good at. I felt that wrestling was a good way to take out these frustrations and fears.

My wrestling career ended up in disastrous fashion. I broke my wrist and never won a single match.

But thanks to wrestling, I discovered running.

My wrestling coach sent the team on training runs, and it was during these runs that I discovered the freedom of running. Running finally made me feel good about myself. The fresh air and long stretches of roads liberated me from the brutal teasing I had experienced for years. I decided to run track and cross-country in high school, and despite taking my 2-mile personal best from 14 minutes down to 10:07, I still had competitors look at me at the starting line and say, "You sure aren't built like a runner."

This sentence still sticks with me: "You sure aren't built like a runner."

Nonsense.

If we run, even for a few feet, we are runners—all of us. You've got this book in your hand and have made the commitment to dare to try.

And for that, I consider you a runner.

My story doesn't end with a decent 2-mile time in high school, though. When I was in my thirties, I let my weight go. After I left the army, I stopped running and my equilibrium entailed a lack of physical exercise, drinking beer consistently, and watching TV after I got home from work.

After going through a personal crisis, I decided that I needed to shift my equilibrium and signed up for my first marathon.

It wasn't easy—equilibrium shifts never are.

But after running nearly 4 hours in my debut 26.2 miles, I got hooked and was able to take my personal best down to 2:32 after several years of intense dedication in the form of blood, sweat, and tears. But though I was able to run a fairly competitive personal best, I've never lost touch with the basics of the sport. I've been in your proverbial shoes. I wasn't a state cross-country champion in high school; I didn't earn a college track scholarship; I've never come remotely close to the Olympic track.

I'm one of you.

Chapter 2

LEARN

Before you lace up a pair of trainers for the first time, you will need to know a few things about running. You don't have to become an expert—just a few basics are in order so that you can make some informed decisions about your training. So what exactly does running entail? In order to answer this question, I'd like you to think of the activity in terms of three "Ls": lungs, legs, and laces.

The Lungs

Running is simply moving at a speed faster than a walk so that both of your feet are not on the ground at the same time. In order to do this, you need to apply energy to your body. Your body's bloodstream helps transmit that energy to the muscles. Typically, the energy that allows you to run can come in two forms: oxygenated blood (aerobic) or blood with energy provided without the aid of oxygen (anaerobic). If you've ever sprinted anywhere as fast as possible, you'll probably recall that you weren't able to do it for long. You were most likely keeled over and drawing deep breaths. Your legs were burning and your lungs were on fire. This was anaerobic running. Because of the unrealistic demands placed on it (e.g., "go very fast right now!"), the body didn't have time to provide efficient, oxygenated blood to move the muscles. Instead it needed to get energy from other immediate sources, like the body's glycogen reserves for example, to propel it at a fast rate of speed. By running anaerobic like this, the body creates a nasty waste product (lactate), which ends up causing that burning sensation in the legs you feel when you are sprinting. There are times and places in more advanced running training schedules where anaerobic training can help distance runners, but not in this book. Everything we're going to be dealing with is in the aerobic realm, so that means we want oxygenated blood reaching your muscles, and that oxygen comes from your lungs. So remember to ask yourself this important question when you're training and feeling winded: Am I going anaerobic? If you're wheezing and huffing, you most likely are. All that rapid breathing means your lungs are working hard to get oxygen ASAP to the legs. The lungs can't keep up and so you're going to eventually build up lactate, which is your enemy.

The one takeaway I want you to remember about your lungs is this:

- Don't ever go anaerobic. Monitor your breathing when you are running. If your breathing is pained or strained, SLOW DOWN. Walking is OK. Get your breathing back under control so that you don't build up lactate in your muscles.

The Legs

To run efficiently, you have to have strong legs. And to get a strong pair of legs, you have to run (or walk) repeatedly for a long time, nearly every day. For you, this means doing so for up to 30 minutes a day.

A lot of muscle groups have to work together to propel you down the roads. As a new runner, it's very easy to fall into the trap of becoming obsessed with every little pain that you feel in your legs after your first few runs. Maybe you feel a twinge around your kneecap the next morning after a run or you tighten up in your calves as you finish your 30-minute routine. These pains can lead to worries, and then doubts about your abilities typically follow. You begin to believe you are injured. And once you believe that you are injured, you've begun to break the part of your contract where you agreed to persevere. Note that there may be a time where you will need to be sidelined and will have to temporarily break your contract. Knowing more about your body will help guide you in making this difficult decision. Of all the leg muscles involved in running, there are really three that you should know about:

- **Your calves:** These muscles are located on the back of your lower leg. They pull up your heel to move forward when you run. You need to know about them, because they are typically one of the first muscle groups that cause pain to new runners. Like those lungs of yours, they can also be good indicators of incorrect pace. If you run faster, you are typically up on the balls of your feet, and when you are up on the balls of your feet, you are working those calf muscles harder, so pay attention to them. A certain degree of muscle soreness is normal for new runners, but excessive calf muscle soreness could mean you're going too fast.

- **Your hamstrings:** These are the muscles at the back of the thigh that work to bend and flex the knee. Running requires constant knee movement, so this means your hamstrings are constantly working (in tandem with another muscle, the quadriceps). These are important muscles for you, the 30-minute runner, because they can be the first thing to side-line you. Underdeveloped hamstrings combined with sudden movement (as in a rapid surge of pace or a sudden stop after a sprint) can cause a painful hamstring strain, which is a quick way to terminate your 30-minute contract. Hamstring strains can be avoided by applying the principles of gradualism in training. We will get to that in more detail later in Chapter 3 but for now, just remember that the body doesn't welcome a shock. One of the first places a new runner can break down when pace isn't properly managed is in the hamstrings.

- **Your IT band:** You've probably heard of your calves and your hamstrings, but the IT band? This collection of fibrous tissue, called the iliotibial band, is a vital part of the body for runners. The long band of fibers runs from your pelvis to your knee along your outer thigh. It plays an important stabilizing role when you run. You need to be aware of the IT band, because it's one of the first problem areas that can flare up when you've been running too much too soon (overtraining). Typically, the band gets sore on the outside of the knee. If you've ever heard the term "runner's knee" to describe an injury, that's usually the IT band. Other than knowing that it exists and that it can flare up, you need to be assured that "runner's knee" problems are common in new runners, so if you experience outer-knee

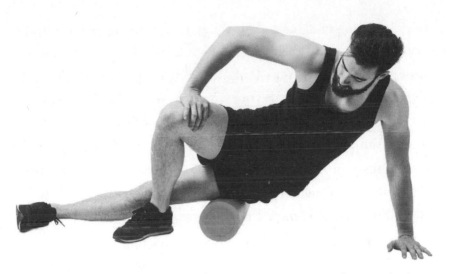

Your IT band plays a key role in running stabilization and can be stretched. Photo courtesy of iStock/panic_attack

soreness and light pain after running, you most likely have an inflamed IT band. The good news is that there are stretches and other ways to recover from IT band syndrome that I'll share with you in Chapters 3 and 6.

The one takeaway I want you to remember about your legs is this:

- Runners need strong legs to ward off injury. Strong legs take time to develop, so it's important to pay attention to three parts of the leg as you are starting out: your calves, hamstrings, and IT band. These areas are especially vulnerable to injury in new runners.

The Laces

When you imagine yourself running, you close your eyes and picture the open road ahead of you. You do a quick "system check" of your body and realize that you've got your pace under control. You know that, because your breathing isn't strained; you aren't wheezing. Your lungs are delivering copious amounts of that precious oxygen to your muscles. You know from reading this chapter that you're right where you need to be: in that sweet aerobic zone. Excellent. Your calves aren't on fire and your hamstrings aren't strained. Your IT band isn't sore. Great. So what else could go wrong? The answer to that question is the one (or two) thing that is literally the closest thing to the roads you are running on: your foot (or feet).

Your foot is a miraculous piece of anatomy. It has twenty-six bones, thirty-three joints, and over one hundred muscles. Yes, there are a lot of things that can go wrong with your actual feet when you're running. You may have heard experienced runners talk about the condition known as plantar fasciitis, which is an inflammation at the bottom of your feet. But foot injuries aren't something I want you concerned about here. Following the advice and schedules in Chapter 3 should prevent you from having to deal with foot-related injury. What I want you to know with regards to your feet can be summarized in one word: pronation.

You may not realize it, but one thing that differentiates runners is how they actually "pronate" when they run. This term refers to how the inside of your foot naturally rolls when your outer heel makes contact with the ground. It rolls as a way to help pass the force of impact to the lower leg, which can handle it better than those twenty-six bones and thirty-three joints can. Your foot's arch usually dictates how much you naturally pronate. Normal pronation is typically a 15 percent roll. Overpronation indicates a larger roll (usually flat-footed runners) and underpronation refers to less of a roll.

There isn't a right or wrong answer to pronation. You are simply one of the three types of pronators based on the size of your arch. *But there is a wrong answer in terms of what type of running shoe you choose to wear.* This is the part that I want to remember: **If you wear a shoe with inadequate support based on your pronation, all sorts of things could go wrong with your running when you are starting out.** The feet help transfer the stresses of contact with the ground, and if those stresses aren't passed efficiently, then muscles and bones are excessively strained. Therefore, the best bet for new runners is to first get their feet analyzed by an expert. Don't worry. This isn't an expensive procedure. It can be as simple as taking an old pair of running or walking shoes into a running store and having an expert who understands pronation examine them and suggest the right kind of shoe for you. Some specialty running stores even have you jog a bit on a treadmill so they can analyze your stride. Once you know how you pronate (under, neutral, over), I want you to write that down in the first page of your training log (see Chapter 3). This is a vital piece of information that can come in handy when we cover stretching in Chapter 6, because different pronation requires different types of preventative treatment to ward off injury.

The one takeaway I want you to remember about your feet is this:

- The size of your arch typically dictates the way your feet come into contact with the ground when you run. This is known as pronation. To support your feet properly, you need to buy the right shoe and know that your pronation can impact your running in other ways.

Chapter 3

TRAIN

You've got your signed contract in hand, you're mindful of the forces of resistance required to shift your equilibrium, and you know a few things about your body.

Now it's time to train.

Before getting too far into it, I want you to remember three training maxims. These should be in your head during all of your workouts and even with you on race day.

- **Training Maxim #1:** <u>Doing something is better than doing nothing</u>. What will follow in this chapter are prescribed workouts to get you started on your 30-minute routine. Remember this—following these schedules to a tee is practically impossible. Life will eventually get in the way of your training. For instance, on a day you are supposed to do a challenging workout, you may be in bed sick with the flu. With that being said, I want you to remember that any exercise is better than no exercise. Putting one foot in front of the other is what counts.

- **Training Maxim #2:** <u>Running isn't a recipe</u>. A common mistake of first-time runners is to get tricked into thinking that running is an exact science. Do exactly what "the book" says, like a recipe, and somehow you will magically transform into the runner on the cover. This won't work. As you start to learn how to run, it's imperative that you learn to become flexible and trust your body. These schedules are to be used as guideposts but are not an absolute. So I'm hereby empowering you to learn to become your own coach. This may seem daunting—especially if you've never run before. And that's OK. The more you run, the more you learn about the sport, your incredible body, and your ability to trust yourself.

- **Training Maxim #3:** <u>You will have good training days and bad training days</u>. Bear in mind that, like a day at work or your relationships with your loved ones, you will simply have good runs and bad runs. There are many reasons why this can be, but don't waste too much time trying to get to the bottom of why a particular run seems harder or easier than another. You may feel terrible on a day where you are supposed to run hard, for example. Many coaches will tell you to "gut through it" and "do the workout no matter what" with a no-pain-no-gain prescription. That's not me. If you feel awful on a day where you are supposed to work out, then ease up. Do what you can, but don't quit. Just put one foot in front of another.

This book isn't going to transform you into an Olympic athlete. It's here to open your eyes to the sport and get you changing your approach to life—shifting the equilibrium from unhealthy to healthy. Be good to yourself when you set out on your new adventure and keep these three training maxims in mind while running.

First Things First: Get a Physical

All of us should be getting routine physicals at our doctor's office. The frequency of these depends on many factors, but before you even lace up one shoe and set out for your first journey on the path towards wellness, you need to schedule an appointment to see a doctor and get a comprehensive physical exam. In the exam, be sure to tell the doctor the following things about yourself specific to running:

- You desire to make positive changes about your health.
- Your intention to begin running (or resume it if you have run before).
- Any concerns you may have about running.
- Your specific running goals.
- Show your doctor your signed 30-Minute Running Contract that you've made with yourself from Chapter 1.

Ask your doctor if he/she thinks you are capable of this new undertaking. If not, then understand what his/her concerns are and what steps you need to take to be able to start running. If you've got a green light, then congratulations! Make sure that you let your doctor know that you'd like to check back in with him/her regularly at a time he/she thinks best given what you intend to accomplish in the next three months. Hopefully, during your physical, you will get some basic diagnostics about your health such as weight, resting heart rate, blood pressure, and cholesterol levels. Ask for this information so that you can add it to your training log.

Your Training Log

Keeping a record of your training is imperative. A good log can be used to help you understand patterns in your training. It also acts as a way for you to see what's coming your way so that you can mentally prepare. A log also can serve as a diary where you can enter free-form commentary about your feelings to help you get in better touch with your body.

Your training log can be a simple blank calendar or diary with the days of the week listed on each page. You don't need to buy a fancy running journal. Just use paper or something equivalent online. This piece of "equipment" will serve as both your "headlights" (you'll write out your full training schedule in it) and your "rear-view mirror" (you'll be expressing how you feel during your workouts) during your running journey.

At a minimum your log needs to have the following elements:

- Daily schedule for the duration of the training plan. Make sure you list your weekly purpose for each training week.
- Transfer over any diagnostic health information that you received from your doctor's office after your physical (resting heart rate, cholesterol levels, and blood pressure).
- Next to each week, write down your current weight. Make sure you weigh yourself before you begin your training schedule and then once a week, on the same day of the week, thereafter. Also try to weigh yourself at approximately the same time of day (preferably once you wake up with no clothes on, perhaps before you take a shower) so that you have an apples-to-apples comparison point. If you are able to keep up

with the schedule and improve how you eat, you should see a reduction in your weight over time, which can be a tremendous motivating factor.

- On each calendar day in your log, write out the following:
  - **What you were supposed to be doing that day according to your training plan.** A week before you begin training, consult your log and add the forecasted temperature and wind speed/direction. By knowing what weather conditions you may face, you can plan your wardrobe and your route. For example, if it's supposed to snow on a day that you are to run steady for 30 minutes, the longest period of time prescribed in this book, you can ensure you select a more forgiving, less hilly route, because the snow itself will be enough of a challenge for you. When I was a logistics officer in the army, we often used a phrase that's applicable here. We called it the seven Ps: "Proper Prior Planning Prevents Piss-Poor Performance."
  - **What you ended up doing on that day.**
  - **The day's temperature when you departed on your run.**
  - **The wind speed and direction.**
  - **How you felt (free-form journaling).** If you experienced any doubts or pains. Conversely, make sure you write out days that you felt strong and confident.
  - **Any relevant info on your diet and hydration such as if you tried a new healthy meal.**
  - **Your sleep pattern for the night before.**
  - **If you purchase new running shoes, go ahead and log that as a specific entry so that you can track in subsequent entries how much wear and tear you are accumulating on the shoes.**

- **If you are completing your 5K, make sure you log the time you completed so you know how it compares against previous personal-best times.**

A good log is a detailed one with a lot of annotations. It will help you establish patterns that can help you prevent injury and understand why you may be feeling a certain way. For example, if you noticed that you were bored on certain days, it may have to do with the fact that you ran the same course, so pick a new one. Use these logs as pieces of evidence that can also help guide you to draw conclusions and form patterns about your training. You may notice that you're improving and getting stronger. A route you used to cover in 20 minutes, you can now cover in 15. This kind of written feedback should help you see real progress and bolster your morale.

The Training Schedules

You've arrived at the heart of the book: the actual workouts you will be doing. Note that there are three daily schedules for the 5K distance in this book. Before you flip to the right schedule for you, understand that each schedule uses the same three daily principles, which are as follows:

- **Intensity:** This is given in terms of "Easy," "Medium," or "Hard."
- **Workout type:** This is what you are supposed to be doing on that specific day.
- **Duration:** This is a number by which you will be abiding for your particular workout. For cross-training days, the number could be repetitions or time in seconds. For hills and speed work, the number could be repetition of hills or laps to run.

So an example day in the schedule could look like this:

Day 2: Tuesday: Easy, Walk, 20. This means that the second day of your schedule, a Tuesday, is an easy day and that you are to walk for 20 minutes.

Every schedule includes the same six types of workouts:

- **Walk**
- **Walk/Run**
- **Steady Running**
- **Hills**
- **Speed Work**
- **Rest or Cross-Train**

I've spelled out these types, because in order for you to progress as a runner, you need to be able to train different parts of your body and, most importantly, to make sure that you are able to rest and recover appropriately so that you can stay healthy and avoid injury. Below are detailed descriptions of these workout types broken down into what they are, why they are important, and what pitfalls you should avoid:

- **Walking: Easy-Intensity Workout**
  - **What it is:** Going outside and taking a walk. No, that isn't a simplification. A book about beginner running actually prescribes a decent amount of walking. If you've never run before, you need to condition your body accordingly, and the best way to do that is to take walks.
  - **Why it's important:** Walking is an excellent way to strengthen the ligaments and tendons in your legs without the physical stress of applying excess weight to them that you encounter in running. Walking also can elevate your heart rate and this leads, over time, to improved

circulation, which means your body becomes more efficient and can, in theory, run faster. It can also burn a lot of calories, and the more pounds you can shed before you take on running, the less weight you'll have to bear during your first 5K. And there's one more benefit of a walk: peace of mind. Getting out the door, breathing in some fresh air, and listening to the birds chirping is good for your mind. Plan ahead for your walks, and choose a good route in advance. If you're not sure how far you need to go to cover a particular amount of time, then do an "out and back," which means setting an alarm on your watch or smartphone for half the time you are supposed to walk and turn around when you reach that time. The more you walk, the more you will learn about your route. A good rule of thumb for walking is approximately 3 miles per hour, so if you need to walk for 30 minutes, then look for routes that measure 1.5 miles in distance. Vary your walk routes, too. As you gain experience, don't be afraid to branch out around your home. If you live near a nice park or trail network, head there for some added serenity.

- **Pitfalls to avoid:** Don't "speed walk." Your pace for these workouts should be totally relaxed. Also, don't get into the habit of "racing" against yourself on your routes. If you covered a particular walking route in 20 minutes one day, don't try to "beat" that time. Also, along those lines, make sure you walk for the entire time as prescribed in the schedule.
- **Walk/Run: Medium-Intensity Workout**
  - **What it is:** Walking for a specific amount of time and then running for a specific amount of time. The amount

of time that you will walk and run is bracketed in the schedule in time walking/time running. An example on the training schedule would look like this: **Day 9: Tuesday: Medium, Walk/Run, 20 (4/1)**. This example means that on the ninth day of your schedule, a Tuesday, you are doing a medium-level intensity workout, a walk/ run for 20 minutes. The 4/1 means that you will walk four minutes and then run for one minute. Then run for four minutes, then walk for one minute until your 20 minutes are up. You'll notice that the beginning days of the schedule has the most time spent walking and little spent running. As the schedule progresses, the time you are to spend running increases slightly so that your body slowly adjusts to this awesome new endeavor.

- **Why it's important:** The body doesn't ever respond well to a sudden shock. If you've never run before, then the best way to learn how to do it is in small doses, as this kind of exertion on a beginner's body can cause significant stress. I consider the walk/run to be the single-most important workout in the entire book. If you can learn to master the art of the walk/run, solidifying the amount of time you spend walking while increasing your running time, then ultimately you will be able to cover the entire 5K distance on the run.

- **Pitfalls to avoid:** Go easy on yourself. If you can't cover the time that the book prescribes for running, reduce according to how you feel. Remember Training Maxim #1: **something is better than nothing.** So if you can only run for 30 seconds and walk for five minutes when you were supposed to run for one minute and walk for 4.5

minutes, that's perfectly OK. Don't beat yourself up about it. *Do what you can*. Conversely, feel free to experiment with longer running periods than the training schedules if you feel good about it. But the name of the game with this workout is gradualism. Any period of walk/run is a success.

- **Steady Running: Medium-Intensity Workout**
  - **What it is:** Just running, at as slow a pace as you need, in order to cover a specific time period prescribed in the schedule.
  - **Why it's important:** This workout is the logical next step after walk/run. Training to run steady for a certain number of minutes is a way to teach your body to allocate energy accordingly. Additionally, a steady run continues to build on all the nice benefits that walking offers, such as strengthening tendons and ligaments. Consistent running also improves your circulatory system by widening existing blood vessels and creating new ones in your legs, making each successive run easier as more, efficient blood flow translates into less effort required to cover the same distance at the same speed.
  - **Pitfalls to avoid:** Steady running can also mean "easy" running. It shouldn't be hard running where you are struggling to breathe and not sure you will be able to make it. If you have just started doing steady running and feel like you can't make it for the whole time, go ahead and give yourself a break with a walk/run interval or two to see you through the duration of the workout. Also, if your steady running is causing you excessive pain, then stop the workout altogether. Always err on the side of caution.

- **Hills: Hard-Intensity Workout**
  - **What it is:** A series of short-length runs at a faster pace up a hill for a determined number of times as designated in the training schedule. The training schedule will call out the number of hills you should complete and these are typically done after a warmup of a set duration of minutes has been completed and they will end with a cooldown run. The hills are described as "repeats," which means you will repeat climbing the same hill for a set number of repetitions. One hill "repeat" entails running from the bottom to the top and walking or jogging back down to the bottom. Though many advanced runners choose different types of hills to do their workout, the hills that you should plan to run as a beginner should be gently sloped and no more than 400 feet in length. This is a little larger than the average city block.
  - **Why it's important:** There are very few completely flat 5K courses. Accordingly, you should be prepared to tackle some elevation in your training. But besides practicing on hills in preparation for race day, hills are also phenomenal sources to improve your overall fitness. A hill's elevation forces the ankles, legs, and lungs to work harder than they do on a flat surface. Hills also present a mental challenge and doing "repeats" gives you many rewards for reaching the summit.
  - **Pitfalls to avoid:** When you begin your hill workout, think about how you will allocate your energy. Don't go "all out" in the first one or two repeats or else you will have a hard time doing all the repeats. There isn't a rush to get back down the hill, so walk if you want to. In terms

of your form, make sure you aren't hunched too far over. Imagine that a string tied around your waist is pulling at you so that your hips are aligned with your shoulders, forming an imaginary straight line. Don't forget to use your arms to help pump your legs up to the top. If the slope of the hill you've chosen is causing you to breathe too much to summit it, then pick something more forgiving.

- **Speed Work: Hard-Intensity Workout**
  - **<u>What it is</u>:** A series of laps at a faster pace around a track. Like hill workouts, these laps will start with a warmup run and end with a cooldown period. Between your laps, you will be given a length of time that you can rest and recover before doing your next repeat. Most tracks are 400 meters in length, so if I prescribe two laps, then this equates to 800 meters. A little over $4 \times 400m$ laps is one mile. Many running books dole out specific guidelines as to how fast you should be running during your speed work. Given the fact that runners of all abilities could be covering this distance at a different speed, this element of training is typically the hardest to specify. The Internet is full of pace calculators and predictors. The good news is that you don't need to worry about any of this for your speed work. So how fast should you run your "hard" laps? I just want you to concern yourself with two concepts: running at a pace faster than your "steady" lap and paying close attention to your breathing.
    - *Your "steady" lap:* When you show up to the track, I want you to run one lap at a steady pace. This pace should be completely relaxed and effortless.

Remember this time. During the workout itself, the times you should be running for your laps should be faster than this "steady" pace. They don't have to be any faster than one second. Overachieving—running them 5 or more seconds faster than your steady lap—is OK, but be careful and ensure that you can run all the laps you are supposed to run in the hard-intensity workout.

- *Your breathing:* While you are running your workout laps, pay very close attention to how you are breathing. As you've learned in Chapter 1, any time you have to breathe heavily in a run usually means that you are going "anaerobic." Expect this to some degree during your speedier laps, but actively monitor yourself. A good rule of thumb: if you are breathing so much that you couldn't carry on a short conversation with a workout partner then you are probably running too fast. **Very important**—if you ever experience any kind of chest pain, then stop immediately and seek medical attention. While speed work is an important element of training for a 5K, remember that it's not vital for your success as a beginner. If you are struggling doing your speed work, then go easy on yourself and run these laps at a steady pace instead. Also, during your recovery period between fast laps, make sure that your breathing is completely recovered—which means you can carry on a normal conversation with someone without any effort. If you are breathing heavily at the time you are supposed to head out for another faster lap, then take a longer break.

- **<u>Why it's important</u>:** Running at a speed faster than you are comfortable with is a great way to strengthen your legs and increase the flow of blood to your muscles. Think of this momentary discomfort as a vital part of your equilibrium shift. These workouts will leave you tired and require extra mental focus, but the work you put in on the track will pay dividends on race day.

- **<u>Pitfalls to avoid</u>:** Similar to hill repeats, don't go all-out in the first few laps around the track, and make sure it's slightly faster than your first "steady" lap. Use your rest and recovery time to "reset" your focus. Make each lap count. If you are to complete these workouts on a hot day, try to do them early in the morning or late in the day so that the heat doesn't make the training harder than it has to be. Remember to err on the side of caution here. These types are workouts aren't easy. You will be pushing yourself but should never be at an extreme level of fatigue.

- **Rest or Cross-Training: Easy-Intensity Workout**

  - **<u>What it is</u>:** This element of training entails no running or walking. Some days you will be given absolutely nothing to do (rest), and other days the task will involve cross-training. Rest means you get a day off from working out. This means what it means. It doesn't mean you go for a long walk or hop on an exercise bike. Do no exercise on these days. Enjoy the rest; you deserve the break! Cross-training will be prescribed occasionally to help you pay attention to parts of your body that supplement and support your running, like your core and your arms. Specific cross-training exercises are listed later in this chapter and will be explained in more detail there.

- **<u>Why it's important</u>: Resting your body properly is the most important aspect of training.** Most first-time runners think that pain goes with the territory and so they push themselves excessively. They don't know if the fatigue and pains they feel are normal and so they tend to go all out. This leads, in many cases, to injury or mental burnout. These first-timers grow despondent and end up giving up on the sport forever—insistent that they just aren't cut out to be a runner. This is why resting matters so much. A body at rest after the right level of exertion is a good thing. The heart slows down and gently pushes blood through the capillaries, allowing any torn muscle fibers to repair/grow and any waste products in the blood, like lactic acid, to exit the body. First-timers will be given a lot of rest/breaks early in their schedule to allow for the body to transition at the proper pace.

- **<u>Pitfalls to avoid</u>:** Eager beginners tend to view rest and recovery days as "bad" or even "wasted." They resist resting, because they think they can push their bodies to run faster. Don't fall into this trap. Just because you enter a rest/recovery day feeling fantastic does not give you the license to skip it. Additionally, as they start to get a few solid weeks of training under them, beginners can gain a sense of invincibility. They are through the difficult periods of the equilibrium shift. Their bodies are changing for the better. They feel stronger and so they think they can therefore work out five or more days a week. Rest is for the weak, right? No! Even world-class runners take days off. You can, too.

Weekly Purpose

Along with a daily workout, you will notice that your training schedule spells out a weekly purpose. The three types of weekly purposes are as follows:

- **Rest and Recover**
- **Base Building**
- **Hills or Speed Work**

This "macro" level of detail should be helpful for you if you end up needing to alter a specific training day. For example, Week 5 of the schedule has a purpose listed as "Hills/Speed Work." If you ended up travelling for work to a location with no hills or a track near you, you could perhaps adjust your workouts until you return to a better-suited location. Another example is if your week's purpose is to "Rest and Recover" and the schedule has you doing some light recovery running, but you feel just plain awful, then go ahead and skip the run altogether. Note that "Rest and Recover" weeks do call for some running in order to help keep the body active and the mind fresh.

"Base Building" is a running term that is similar to the "steady" runs you are doing throughout the week. Building a base entails running or walking simply to strengthen your legs, lungs, and mind. Think of this weekly purpose as laying the "foundation" for your proverbial "house" (your body). A good structural foundation contains a lot of concrete and rebar in order to withstand the forces of nature like earthquakes, wind, and snow. These weeks typically appear early in your schedule and will serve to build you up so that you can withstand faster hill and speed work as well as the actual challenges that appear on the day of your first 5K.

Without a good foundation, it will be more difficult to run faster. Also, the better your "base," the easier you can ward off injury.

Cross-Training for Beginners

Some days in your schedule, you will be prescribed cross-training exercises. Oftentimes, runners who are beginning their training focus on everything below the waist, but neglect their upper body.

This is unfortunate.

Running is entirely an all-body endeavor. The next time you are out for a run, take inventory of what parts are in motion. Your legs are propelled thanks to your arms. Every swing of the arm means all the muscles in that part of the body are in play and if a muscle is being used, it should be trained and monitored. A more complex example of this all body concept is what happens in your "core." Think of the core as all the muscles that comprise your torso (stomach, back, and hips). All of these muscles are required to help you put one foot in front of the other, and to do it faster, they need to be strong, healthy, and working in harmony. Running alone can strengthen your core, but all these additional muscles could use some extra work, which is why there are some days on your schedule where you will work on them doing three basic exercises: Planks, Standing Bicycle Crunches, and Burpees. In your schedule, each day of cross-training will specify the exercise and the number of repetitions you should be doing. What follows below are specific details on how to complete these exercises, broken out into what part of the body the exercise works, how to complete the exercise (in steps), and dos/don'ts to adhere to as you complete the exercise.

The Plank

What it works: This is a phenomenal simple workout for your entire core and other areas of your upper torso. The Plank specifically works your abdominals, arms, lower back, and shoulders.

How to do it:

Step 1: Find a soft mat or stretch of carpeted floor and get into the push-up position.

Step 2: Bend your arms at 90-degree angles and bring them down so that your forearms rest on the floor while you are up on the balls of your feet.

Step 3: Start your watch and hold that position for the designated time in the schedule.

Dos and Don'ts:

Do: If you've never done these before, then cut yourself a break and put your knees on the ground to support you. As you gain

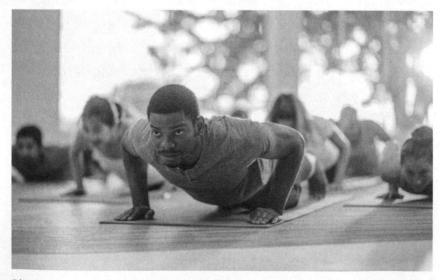

Planking is a simple, yet effective exercise that works a wide range of muscles at the same time. Photo courtesy of iStock/FatCamera

strength and feel confident, try to lift your knees off the ground and support your weight only on your forearms and toes. You can also do more advanced variations of the plank that involve lifting a foot or hand to work different angles of your muscles. Keep a record of your longest plank as a fun way to compete against yourself to see if you can break it.

Don't: Let your back sag. As you tire, this will be the first thing you will want to do. It's better to go to your knees than have your stomach dip down towards the floor. Ensure your body forms a straight line from head to the feet. Also, don't despair if you have a hard time with this initially. The more you do it the stronger you will become. Finally, don't forget to breathe normally throughout the exercise.

Standing Bicycle Crunch

What it works: Your oblique abdominals. Most "crunch" exercises are done on the floor laying down and increase the risk of straining your neck and back muscles. The Standing Bicycle Crunch is a much better way for beginners to work the abs.

How to do it:

Step 1:   Stand up with your feet shoulder-width apart. Point your toes forward. Put your hands behind your head like you were to do a sit-up (palms facing out with fingertips touching your head). Take a deep breath.

Step 2:   Raise your right knee up and bring it across your body so that it touches your left elbow. Exhale.

Step 3:   Repeat with the opposite leg and elbow.

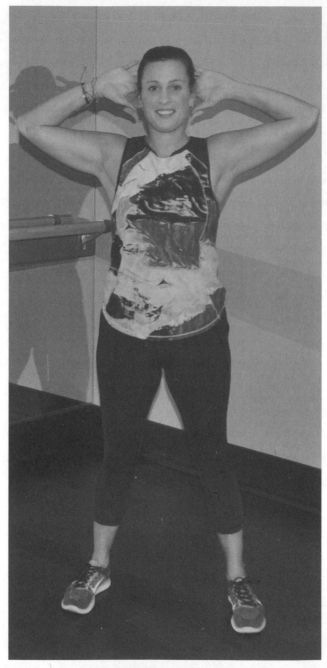

Remember to stand with your feet shoulder-width apart when you begin the Standing Bicycle Crunch.
Model credit: Meredith Turk Wright

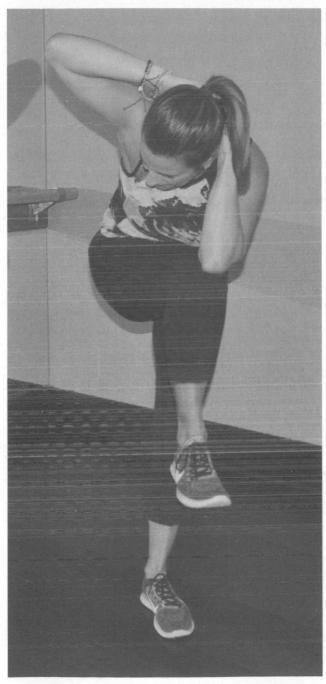

Touch your elbow to your opposite knee and exhale.
Model credit: Meredith Turk Wright

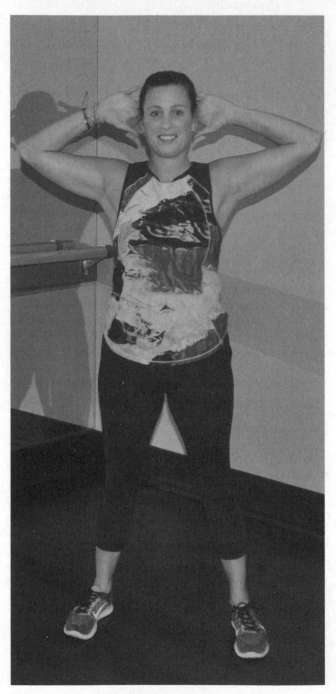

Return to the start position.
Model credit: Meredith Turk Wright

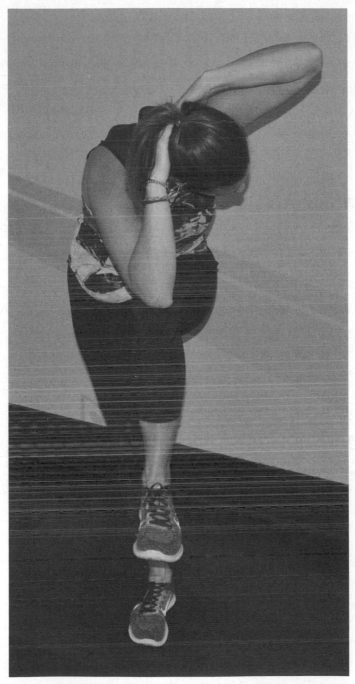

Repeat the exercise with the opposite knee and elbow.
Model credit: Meredith Turk Wright

Dos and Don'ts:

Do: If this is a new exercise to you, then it may be really hard to keep your balance. Go ahead and place one hand on a wall for support. Also, bring your elbow and your knee as close as you can to one another. They don't have to touch. Do what you can. Make sure you are breathing properly through the crunch. As a variation, you can perform all repetitions on one side before switching to the other side.

Don't: Go fast. This isn't a race. Take your time and go slow. The faster you speed through it, the more you are cheating your body by using gravity and momentum.

Burpees

What it works: This exercise is also called a "squat thrust" and is typically performed in four steps. It's a fantastic way to work your upper body and core. It also gets your heart rate up.

How to do it:

Step 1: Find a mat or a large carpeted area and begin in the standing position with feet shoulder-width apart. Bend at the hips and try to touch the floor, with the palms of your hands facing forward, in the squat position.

Step 2: Kick your feet back onto the push-up position.

Step 3: Kick your feet back to the squat position.

Step 4: Stand up.

Dos and Don'ts:

Do: If you are worried about kicking your feet out and in during Steps 2 and 3 then it's OK to walk them back slowly. If you're looking for more of a challenge, do a push-up after Step 2

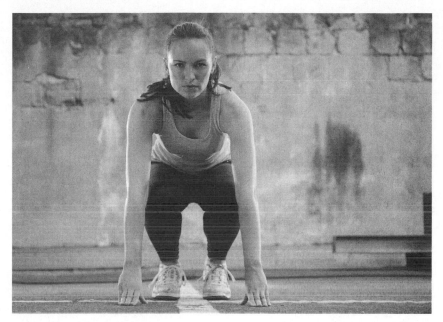

Remember that the burpee isn't a race. Take your time and do the steps using good form and focus. Photo courtesy of iStock.com/Thomas_EyeDesign

(going to your knees is OK), and you can also jump up in the air with your hands reaching skyward after Step 4.

Don't: Rush through the steps. It's not about doing them as quickly as possible. Be methodical and don't forget to breathe through the steps. Make sure your torso is aligned with your head while you are kicking your feet out and back, as it can be easy to become crooked.

Other Ways to Cross-Train

There are just three exercises in this book. I intentionally made things very simple, because I believe these work the right muscles you need to supplement your running. However, there are many other things you can do. If you've never worked out before and lack the confidence to try other body-weight exercises on your own, I would caution you to not do anything else. Stay away from the body-building and fitness websites, because you may end up doing something that gets you injured.

But I do think you can supplement these exercises on your cross-training days in the schedule by doing other things that burn calories in a low-impact way. Here are a few example cross-training exercises that you have a green light from me to experiment with.

- **Swimming.** This is a phenomenal low-impact exercise that burns a ton of calories while getting your heart rate up. Any swimming is fine. Like running, try to follow the 30-minute-max principle. If you're not a good swimmer, then find a pool you can wade in and walk "laps" for 10 to 30 minutes.

- **Gardening.** Most people don't consider this to be a "cross-training" sport, but if you've ever planted a garden, then you'll know that it requires quite a bit of lifting, walking, and bending.

- **Biking.** If you own a bike, dust it off and go for a 20- to 30-minute ride on your cross-training days. Cycling is similar to swimming in that it's a low-impact alternative to work your leg muscles, increasing the flow of blood to your capillaries and helping flush that nasty lactic acid that builds up when you've been running hard.

- **Yoga.** The spiritual practice is an outstanding way to stretch your body and be at peace after a difficult running week. This form of exercise is gaining in popularity, so if you've never tried it before, there are certainly clinics near where you live that you can attend to give yoga a try.

- **Meditation.** This isn't cross-training for your body—rather cross-training for your mind. The act of running, especially during difficult workouts, can sometimes seem jarring, so it's good to balance this disruption by grounding yourself with quiet serenity. Know that there is no right or wrong way to meditate. If you've never tried it before, then follow this simple routine. You'll find that you will have the most success meditating in the early morning or before you go to bed.

- Find the quietest room in your house. If you don't have one, go to a park or nature preserve with a comfortable patch of grass where you can hear only the sounds of nature.
- If you are in a room, turn the lights off and close the shades/draw the curtains.
- Light a candle.
- Sit on the floor or on a mat in a comfortable position. You don't need to assume the traditional "lotus pose" that stereotypically is ascribed to meditation. You can sit cross-legged or however you feel the most at ease.
- Close your eyes.
- Take one deep breath, pause for a second, and exhale slowly. As you exhale, imagine the stress and strain of your training as well as your life's other troubles leaving your body.
- When you breathe in, imagine that you are breathing in peace and strength.
- Continue this breathing pattern for a few minutes.
- When you feel ready, lie down on the mat and close your eyes. Stop your meditation by blowing out the candle and gradually allow light to return to your room by opening the shades—don't immediately turn on the light.

The Training Schedules

All of the schedules contain the same elements of training as described in this chapter, but vary in terms of difficulty. Note that, in keeping with the principles of the book, no single run or workout for the 5K plan will exceed 30 minutes. If you're unsure which schedule is best for you, choose the easier schedule, at least at the beginning.

Workout Type Table

Workout Type	Intensity	Description	Example
Rest or Cross-Train	Easy	Either no working out at all (Rest) or Cross-Training, to build strength and stamina in different parts of your body to supplement your running and prevent injury.	Cross-Train • 3 × 20 Standing Bicycle Crunches • 3 × Plank (45 seconds) • 10 Burpees This means do three repetitions of 20 Standing Bicycle Crunches, three sets of The Plank for 45 secs, and then 10 Burpees on this day for your workout.
Walk	Easy	A relaxed-pace outdoor walk.	Easy, Walk, 20. This means walk for 20 minutes.
Walk/Run	Medium	A mixture of walking and running, given in total number of minutes to walk and run.	Medium Walk/Run 20 (5/1). This means walk for five minutes, then run for one minute for a total of 20 minutes.
Steady Running	Medium	Just running, at as slow a pace as you need, in order to cover a specific time period prescribed in the schedule.	Medium, Steady Running, 10. This means do steady running for 10 minutes straight.

(Continued)

Workout Type	Intensity	Description	Example
Hills	Hard	Running up a hill and then jog or walk back down in a number of repetitions.	Hard, Hills • 10 minutes, Walk • 3 Hills • 5-minute Cooldown This means do 10 minutes of Walking, then do three Hill repetitions, and finally do five minutes of Cooldown (walk or run).
Speed Work	Hard	A series of fast laps around the track with rest between laps.	Hard, Speed Work • 5 minutes, Walk • 1 Steady lap • 2 Hard laps with 3 minutes Rest between • 5-minute Cooldown This means do five minutes of Walking then one lap at a Steady lap. Then do one Hard lap (faster than your Steady lap) with three minutes of Rest, then one more lap around the track and a 5-minute Cooldown (walk or run).

Weekly Purpose Table

Purpose Type	Description
Rest and Recover	In this week, you are giving your body a break after a longer period of hard weeks before it. This week will help you ensure you recover your energy and allow your muscles to rest so that you can build in subsequent weeks and minimize the risk of injury.
Base Building	This week is all about building muscular strength and endurance so that you can run longer and faster. Think of it as laying the right, solid foundation that you can build on in subsequent weeks with Hills or Speed Work.
Hills or Speed Work	Typically these are your hardest weeks where you will be running faster and with more intensity in the other two weeks.

The Three Training Maxims to Memorize

Training Maxim #1	Doing something is better than doing nothing.
Training Maxim #2	Running isn't a recipe.
Training Maxim #3	You will have good training days and you will have bad training days.

Training Schedule 1

Follow this schedule if you've never run before. You just want to complete a 5K either by walking or running it.

Week 1's Purpose: Base Building

Mon	Tues	Wed	Thurs	Fri	Sat	Sun
Easy, Walk, 5	Rest	Easy, Walk, 10	Rest	Easy, Walk, 15	Rest	Easy, Walk, 15

Week 2's Purpose: Base Building

Mon	Tues	Wed	Thurs	Fri	Sat	Sun
Rest	Easy, Walk, 20	Rest	Easy, Walk, 10	Rest	Easy, Walk, 25	Rest

Week 3's Purpose: Rest and Recover

Mon	Tues	Wed	Thurs	Fri	Sat	Sun
Cross-Train Plank 2 × 30 secs	Rest	Easy, Walk 20	Rest	Easy, Walk, 20	Rest	Cross-Train Plank 3 × 30 secs

Week 4's Purpose: Base Building

Mon	Tues	Wed	Thurs	Fri	Sat	Sun
Rest	Easy, Walk 20	Rest	Easy, Walk 20	Cross-Train Plank 3 × 30 secs	Rest	Easy, Walk 30

Week 5's Purpose: Base Building

Mon	Tues	Wed	Thurs	Fri	Sat	Sun
Rest	Medium, Walk/ Run 15 (4/1)	Rest	Medium, Walk/Run 20 (5/1)	Rest	Easy, Walk, 20	Rest

Week 6's Purpose: Hills or Speed Work

Mon	Tues	Wed	Thurs	Fri	Sat	Sun
Easy, Walk, 30	Rest	Hard, Hills • 10 minutes, Walk • 3 Hills • 5-minute Cooldown	Rest	Hard, Hills • 10 minutes, Walk • 4 Hills • 5-minute Cooldown	Rest	Easy, Walk, 20

Week 7's Purpose: Hills or Speed Work

Mon	Tues	Wed	Thurs	Fri	Sat	Sun
Easy, Walk, 20	Rest	Hard, Speed Work • 5 minutes, Walk • 1 Steady Lap • 2 Hard Laps with 3-minute rest between • 5-minute Cooldown	Rest	Rest	Easy, Walk, 30	Medium, Walk/ Run, 20 (4/1)

Week 8's Purpose: Rest and Recover

Mon	Tues	Wed	Thurs	Fri	Sat	Sun
Rest	Cross-Train • Plank 3 × 30 secs • Standing Bicycle Crunches 2 × 20	Easy, Walk, 20	Cross-Train • Plank 3 × 30 secs • Standing Bicycle Crunches 2 × 20	Easy, Walk, 20	Rest	Rest

Week 9's Purpose: Base Building

Mon	Tues	Wed	Thurs	Fri	Sat	Sun
Medium, Walk/Run, 20 (4/1)	Rest	Medium, Steady Running, 10	Cross-Train • Standing Bicycle Crunches 3 × 20	Rest	Medium, Walk/Run, 30 (4/1)	Rest

Week 10's Purpose: Base Building

Mon	Tues	Wed	Thurs	Fri	Sat	Sun
Medium, Steady Running, 10	Rest	Medium, Steady Running, 15	Rest	Medium, Walk/ Run, 20 (3/2)	Rest	Easy, Walk, 30

Week 11's Purpose: Hills or Speed Work

Mon	Tues	Wed	Thurs	Fri	Sat	Sun
Rest	Hard, Speed Work • 5 minutes, Walk • 1 Steady lap • 3 Hard laps with 3-minute Rest between • 5-minute Cooldown	Rest	Medium, 15 minutes Steady Running	Rest	Hard, Speed Work • 5 minutes, Walk • 1 Steady lap • 3 Hard laps with 3-minute Rest between • 5-minute Cooldown	Rest

Week 12's Purpose: Rest and Recover

Mon	Tues	Wed	Thurs	Fri	Sat	Sun
Cross-Train • Standing Bicycle Crunches 3 × 20 • 10 Burpees	Rest	Easy, Walk, 20	Rest	Easy, Walk, 20	Rest	Race Day!

Training Schedule 2

Do this schedule if you've run before but have never run or walked a 5K.

Week 1's Purpose: Base Building

Mon	Tues	Wed	Thurs	Fri	Sat	Sun
Easy, Walk, 10	Rest	Easy, Walk, 15	Rest	Easy, Walk, 15	Rest	Easy, Walk, 20

Week 2's Purpose: Base Building

Mon	Tues	Wed	Thurs	Fri	Sat	Sun
Rest	Easy, Walk, 30	Rest	Easy, Walk, 20	Rest	Easy, Walk, 30	Rest

Week 3's Purpose: Rest and Recover

Mon	Tues	Wed	Thurs	Fri	Sat	Sun
Cross-Train • Plank 2 × 30 secs • Standing Bicycle Crunches 2 × 10	Rest	Easy, Walk, 30	Rest	Easy, Walk, 30	Rest	Cross-Train • Plank 3 × 30 secs • Standing Bicycle Crunches 2 × 10

Week 4's Purpose: Base Building

Mon	Tues	Wed	Thurs	Fri	Sat	Sun
Rest	Medium, Walk/Run, 15 (4/1)	Rest	Easy, Walk, 30	Medium, Walk/Run, 25 (4/1)	Rest	Easy, Walk, 30

Week 5's Purpose: Base Building

Mon	Tues	Wed	Thurs	Fri	Sat	Sun
Rest	Medium, Walk/Run, 30 (4/1)	Rest	Medium, Walk/Run, 20 (3/2)	Rest	Easy, Walk, 30	Rest

Week 6's Purpose: Hills or Speed Work

Mon	Tues	Wed	Thurs	Fri	Sat	Sun
Easy, Walk, 30	Rest	Hard, Hills • 10 minutes, Walk • 3 Hills • 5-minute Cooldown	Rest	Hard, Hills • 10 minutes, Walk • 4 Hills • 5-minute Cooldown	Rest	Easy, Walk, 30

Week 7's Purpose: Hills or Speed Work

Mon	Tues	Wed	Thurs	Fri	Sat	Sun
Easy, Walk, 20	Rest	Hard, Speed Work • 5 minutes, Walk • 1 Steady lap • 2 Hard laps with 3-minute Rest between • 5-minute Cooldown	Rest	Rest	Easy, Walk, 30	Medium, Walk/Run, 30 (3/2)

Week 8's Purpose: Rest and Recover

Mon	Tues	Wed	Thurs	Fri	Sat	Sun
Rest	Cross-Train, • Plank 3 × 30 secs • Standing Bicycle Crunches 2 × 20 • Burpees 2 × 5	Easy, Walk, 30	Cross-Train • Plank 3 × 30 secs • Standing Bicycle Crunches 2 × 20 • Burpees 2 × 5	Easy, Walk, 30	Rest	Rest

Week 9's Purpose: Base Building

Mon	Tues	Wed	Thurs	Fri	Sat	Sun
Medium, Steady Running, 10	Rest	Medium, Steady Running, 20	Cross-Train • Standing Bicycle Crunches 3 × 20 • 8 Burpees	Rest	Medium, Steady Running, 30	Rest

Week 10's Purpose: Base Building

Mon	Tues	Wed	Thurs	Fri	Sat	Sun
Medium, Steady Running, 30	Rest	Medium, Steady Running, 30	Rest	Medium, Steady Running 30	Rest	Easy, Walk, 30

Week 11's Purpose: Hills or Speed Work

Mon	Tues	Wed	Thurs	Fri	Sat	Sun
Rest	Hard, Speed Work • 5 minutes, Walk • 1 Steady lap • 3 Hard laps with 3-minute Rest between • 5-minute Cooldown	Rest	Medium, Steady Running, 30	Rest	Hard, Speed Work • 5 minutes, Walk • 1 Steady lap • 3 Hard laps with 3-minute Rest between • 5-minute Cooldown	Rest

Week 12's Purpose: Rest and Recover

Mon	Tues	Wed	Thurs	Fri	Sat	Sun
Cross-Train • Standing Bicycle Crunches 3 × 20 • Plank 3 × 30 secs • 10 Burpees	Rest	Easy, Walk, 30	Rest	Easy, Walk, 30	Rest	Race Day!

Training Schedule 3

Do this schedule if you've run a 5K before but seek to improve your personal-best time.

Week 1's Purpose: Base Building

Mon	Tues	Wed	Thurs	Fri	Sat	Sun
Easy, Walk, 20	Rest	Easy, Walk, 25	Rest	Easy, Walk, 25	Rest	Easy, Walk, 25

Week 2's Purpose: Base Building

Mon	Tues	Wed	Thurs	Fri	Sat	Sun
Rest	Easy, Walk, 30	Rest	Easy, Walk, 30	Rest	Medium, Walk/ Run, 15 (4/1)	Rest

Week 3's Purpose: Rest and Recover

Mon	Tues	Wed	Thurs	Fri	Sat	Sun
Cross-Train, • Plank 2 × 30 secs • Standing Bicycle Crunches 2 × 10 • 8 Burpees	Rest	Easy, Walk, 30	Rest	Medium, Walk/Run, 20 (4/1)	Rest	Cross-Train, • Plank 3 × 30 secs • Standing Bicycle Crunches 2 × 10 • 8 Burpees

Week 4's Purpose: Base Building

Mon	Tues	Wed	Thurs	Fri	Sat	Sun
Rest	Medium, Walk/ Run, 20 (4/1)	Rest	Easy, Walk, 30	Medium, Walk/ Run, 30 (4/1)	Rest	Easy, Walk, 30

Week 5's Purpose: Base Building

Mon	Tues	Wed	Thurs	Fri	Sat	Sun
Rest	Medium, Steady Running, 20	Rest	Medium, Steady Running, 20	Rest	Medium, Walk/ Run, 30 (3/2)	Rest

Week 6's Purpose: Hills or Speed Work

Mon	Tues	Wed	Thurs	Fri	Sat	Sun
Easy, Walk, 30	Rest	Hard, Hills • 10 minutes, Walk • 3 Hills • 5-minute Cooldown	Rest	Hard, Hills • 5 minutes, Walk • 5 Hills • 5-minute Cooldown	Rest	Easy, Walk, 30

Week 7's Purpose: Hills or Speed Work

Mon	Tues	Wed	Thurs	Fri	Sat	Sun
Medium, Steady Running, 20	Rest	Hard, Speed Work • 5 minutes, Walk • 1 Steady lap • 2 Hard laps with 3-minute Rest between • 5-minute Cooldown	Rest	Rest	Hard, Speed Work • 5 minutes, Walk • 1 Steady lap • 2 Hard laps with 3-minute Rest between • 5-minute Cooldown	Medium, Walk/ Run, 30 (3/2)

Week 8's Purpose: Rest and Recover

Mon	Tues	Wed	Thurs	Fri	Sat	Sun
Rest	Cross-Train • Plank 3 × 30 secs • Standing Bicycle Crunches 3 × 20 • Burpees 2 × 10	Easy, Walk, 30	Cross-Train • Plank 3 × 30 secs • Standing Bicycle Crunches 3 × 20 • Burpees 2 × 10	Medium, Steady Running, 20	Rest	Rest

Week 9's Purpose: Base Building

Mon	Tues	Wed	Thurs	Fri	Sat	Sun
Medium, Steady Running, 30	Rest	Medium, Steady Running, 30	Cross Train • Standing Bicycle Crunches 3 × 20 • 8 Burpees	Rest	Medium, Steady Running, 30	Rest

Week 10's Purpose: Base Building

Mon	Tues	Wed	Thurs	Fri	Sat	Sun
Medium, Steady Running, 30	Rest	Medium, Steady Running, 30	Rest	Medium, Steady Running 30	Rest	Medium, Steady Running, 30

Week 11's Purpose: Hills or Speed Work

Mon	Tues	Wed	Thurs	Fri	Sat	Sun

Rest	Hard, Speed Work
	• 5 minutes, Walk
	• 1 Steady lap
	• 3 Hard laps with
	  3-minute Rest between
	• 5-min Cooldown
		Rest	Medium,
			Steady
			Running,
			30
				Rest	Hard, Speed Work
					• 5 minutes, Walk
					• 1 Steady lap
					• 3 Hard laps with
					  3-minute Rest between
					• 5-min Cooldown
						Medium,
						Steady
						Running,
						30

Week 12's Purpose: Rest and Recover

Mon	Tues	Wed	Thurs	Fri	Sat	Sun
Cross-Train, • Standing Bicycle Crunches, 3 × 20 • Plank 3 × 30 secs • 10 Burpees	Rest	Medium, Steady Running, 20	Rest	Easy, Walk, 30	Rest	Race Day!

Equipment

A common misconception with beginners is that success can come simply by getting all the appropriate gadgets. They attend a pre-race expo and get suckered into buying gear. Don't fall into this trap. To run your first 5K, there are a few essential items that you will absolutely need to buy. There are also other items that might be helpful. Then there are those things that you don't need to waste your money on.

Things you will need to purchase:

- **Running shoes.** Your shoes are the most important piece of gear that you will be purchasing. As you learned in Chapter 2, your stride and natural foot strike can determine the right shoe for you. Instead of detailing all the types of shoes you should consider, it's best to simply go to a pro and ask for help. I strongly recommend that you NOT skimp on your running shoes. Don't buy them online or at a discount chain store. Instead, find a locally-owned running store that has a shoe expert. Be honest with them. Tell them you need help. Explain your concerns. Have them analyze your stride and foot strike, and defer to them. Know that a good pair of shoes typically costs over $100, and don't try to penny-pinch here. Running shoes aren't penny loafers, so they usually don't need to be "broken in." If you experience discomfort during your first run after purchasing them, you probably need to go back to the store and tell your new expert friend how you feel. Also, don't panic if your expert puts you in shoes half a size bigger than what you typically wear. Training shoes need to be slightly bigger to account for the movement of the foot so as to prevent blistering and numbing of the toes. In terms of durability, a good rule of thumb for most running shoes is 300 to 500 miles before you need to replace them. The training schedules in this book all last 12 weeks and, given that you are doing max 30 minutes a day of running, you most likely will not need to purchase new shoes for the duration of the plan.

- **Compression shorts.** As a beginner, you have to prepare for the unfortunate fact that your body is going to rub together in places you never realized was possible. The biggest problem area of chafing is usually between your thighs. Chafing is incredibly painful–especially once heat and sweat kick in. If not treated or prevented, chafing can sideline your running indefinitely. A pair of compression shorts will help ward off this preventable injury.

- **A basic digital watch.** This is entirely a time-based running book. As such, all you need to measure your runs is a watch that comes with a stop/start button and a countdown timer. You don't need to run with a smartphone that tracks your distance, but if you want to bring one for safety purposes, by all means do so. Don't bother tracking, though, and obsessing about how far you've run. It's best to minimize your dependency on technology.

- **Running hat.** Any baseball cap with a brim will do, but it might be worth your money investing in a special running hat, which is typically made from lighter fabric to help keep your head cool.

- **Refillable water bottle.** As a beginner, you need to be hydrating on your walks and runs early in your training schedule. Find a bottle that you don't mind carrying for 30 minutes. Some specialized running water bottles form fit into your hand. I don't think you have to buy these. You can run just as well with a small refillable bottle that has a tight-fitting lid.

- **Band-Aids or moleskin.** These are great to help prevent excessive chafing on smaller parts of your body.

- **For winter running, thin layers of long sleeved shirts, running tights, a knit cap, and gloves.** If you are going to be running in below-freezing temperatures, it's well worth the investment to purchase running tights that can help prevent chafing as well as keep your legs warm. You don't have to spend a lot of money for the other parts of your winter wardrobe, though. In fact, you can purchase lightweight gloves and knit caps at a dollar store. And you can find inexpensive long-sleeved workout shirts at discount chain stores like Target or Old Navy. A supercheap clothing option is Goodwill or the Salvation Army. Remember that you're working out, not dressing up for a fashion show. Comfort matters most.

- **A few cheap bags of frozen peas.** The next time you are at the grocery store, pick up some bags of peas. These aren't to eat, but rather are a cheap way to ice your body. Frozen peas can be excellent reusable ice packs for stiff, swollen, and sore limbs. The small peas will wrap around your legs or feet, forming a nice "ice blanket." When you are done with them, refreeze them.
- **'Attaboy'/'attagirl' rewards.** Consider purchasing little treats that you can "bribe" yourself with if you successfully complete tough workouts or not quit your runs. One idea is to purchase a bunch of gift cards from your favorite restaurants or stores and tape them to a calendar so that you can see them at all times.

Things you might consider buying:

- **An extra pair of running shoes.** Once you find the right kind of shoe, it might be a good idea to purchase an additional pair of the same kind. You can then alternate pairs between workouts. If you buy the same type of shoe, write a #1 and a #2 somewhere on the inside of each pair to remember which shoes go together.
- **Exercise mat.** You can do all the cross-training workouts in this book on a carpeted floor, but it might be more comfortable doing them on a mat. You can find cheap exercise mats in discount stores for as little as $5.
- **Sunglasses.** Squinting can distract you especially on your difficult workout days. Pick a pair of shades that is made for runners. When you find the right kind, ask the salesperson if you have the option to return them if they don't feel comfortable after a run or two.
- **Running belt.** If you need to carry your smartphone with you or don't like running with a bottle of water in your hands, then consider picking up one of these.

<u>Things you probably don't need to buy in order to run your first 5K:</u>

- **A gym membership.** Every exercise and workout prescribed in this book can be done either out on the trails or roads.
- **A treadmill.** There's nothing wrong with treadmills, but there should be enough options in this book for you to get outside and do your workouts in the fresh air as opposed to confined in a gym or home.
- **A smart watch or GPS.** You don't need to know how far your runs are. In fact, I would advise against this. A typical mistake for first-time runners is to become beholden to all the biometric and other data that can be accumulated thanks to all this new lightweight technology that we can get our hands on these days. Usually, the more you know about your run, the more time you spend trying to analyze it and the more likely you are to get caught up worrying if you are running a prescribed distance fast enough.
- **Heart rate monitors.** These devices are for advanced training and can cause confusion for first-time runners. They can also be misleading and oftentimes malfunction. Save your money; don't buy one.
- **Weights.** All the cross-training exercises in this book use your own body weight, so you don't need to buy dumbbells or an expensive weight bench.

Nutrition and Hydration

I'm not a professional nutritionist, so I won't be doling out much dietary advice in this chapter. If you're overweight, your best bet is to pick up a copy of Dr. Michael Moreno's bestselling *The 17*

Day Diet and use that excellent jump-start diet in tandem with the workouts prescribed in this book.

However, there are still some basic nutritional principles that all runners should be adhering to. And regardless whether or not you are overweight, you still should be taking to heart these key concepts:

1. **Refuel and rehydrate after a hard workout or a long, steady run.** If you've done any exercise for 30 minutes, then you need to eat and drink approximately one hour after you've stopped working out. Your body's liver and glycogen stores are most likely depleted. Refuel with a good balance of carbohydrates and protein. Some example refuel options include a bagel, banana, peanut butter and jelly sandwich, or even a large glass of chocolate milk. Supplement this with two large glasses of water or a sports drink of your choice.

2. **Watch the late-night snacking.** Even though you're working out now, you should try to reduce caloric consumption after dinner. Your body will most likely convert these calories to fat. Be mindful of late-evening cravings. If you are hungry at night, drink a tall glass of water, and if that doesn't help, then try one glass of nonfat milk to help ward off the hunger pains. Another way to deal with overeating at the wrong times is to tell yourself that you will try to "savor every bite." This means, especially if you are ravenous, to consciously eat slower. If you are at a meal with friends or family, try to have a conversation with them between your bites. Pace your meals the same way you would pace your runs.

3. **Plan your meals to benefit your runs.** In other words, don't eat a huge lunch before you head out to do your workout. If you're a morning person, consider a light breakfast like a piece

of toast with honey and some coffee about one to two hours before your run. If you run after work, have a light postlunch snack like a granola bar an hour before you hit the roads.

4. **Stay continually hydrated by becoming an expert urine monitor.** I know, it sounds gross, but you should always pay attention to the color of your pee. Typically, the darker it is the more you need to drink. Carry a water bottle around with you at work and sip from it routinely.

5. **Bring water to your hard workouts.** If you are doing track workouts or running up hills, always bring water with you. Take small sips between laps or repeats. If you experience cramping from this, then bring a washcloth and a cooler filled with ice that you can use to dampen your forehead during your recovery period.

6. **Just because it's cold outside doesn't mean you shouldn't drink water.** Your body can become dehydrated even in the winter, so just because you aren't feeling warm on your runs doesn't mean you should cut back on how much water you drink.

7. **Commit to making significant nutritional changes.** Don't let all this hard work go to waste by feeding your strengthening body with garbage. Nutrition and running go hand in hand. They are the one-two punch you need to affect positive change in your life. It's not a cliché that "you are what you eat." Think about your running nutrition as a vital component of your equilibrium shift. Your body operates optimally on a combination of carbohydrates, protein, and fats (CPF). A good rule of thumb for consumption for runners is approximately 70 percent carbs, 20 percent protein, and 10 percent healthy fat (poly- and monounsaturated, NOT saturated fat). Take a moment to think about how you get your CPF.

Ask yourself what choices you make—what are your staple, go-to foods? What follows is an example food substitution table. Create your own and put it on your fridge to use both as a reminder every time you go into the kitchen and as a continual grocery list you can use. Continue to update your substitution lists as you experiment with new healthier foods that you've never considered before.

Food Type	Unhealthy	Healthier
Carbohydrate sources	Sugary snacks, chips, sodas, white bread, candy, cookies	Fruits and green vegetables
Protein sources	Red meat (beef)	Leaner meats like turkey, yogurt, quinoa, beans, soy, hard-boiled eggs
Fat sources	Whole milk, cheese, sausage, fried eggs	Nuts, avocado, skim milk

You can also create a meal-substitution table, using the healthier ingredients, and post it next to your food substitution table to aid you in your weekly meal planning and grocery shopping. Another thing to consider besides the choices you make in your diet is how much you eat. Portion control is essential, especially if you are overweight as you start your training. A few good rules of thumb to follow are to avoid seconds, eat your meals on smaller plates, fill your stomach with veggies instead of bad carbs, and, above all, slow down when you eat. Savor each bite and try dining with friends or family instead of alone.

8. **Shop for your groceries on the edges of the store.** Most grocery stores are designed in similar fashion. The fresh

produce—fruits and vegetables—can be found along the outside aisles of the store. On the inside are the "bad" things for you—unhealthy snacks, like candy and sodas. Not only should you be altering what you eat, but also where you find what you eat. Resist the temptation to get drawn into the middle of the grocery store.

9. **Be careful about overhydrating.** Many first-time runners are so concerned about dehydration that they end up drinking too much water. This can lead to a dangerous condition known as hyponatremia, or water intoxication, where the sodium content in the blood is so diluted, you can become dizzy, cramp up, and, even in serious cases, go into seizure or a coma. A good rule of thumb is to be in touch with your body's fluid levels (by monitoring your urine's color and volume from Tip #4) and drink to your thirst. After your run, replace the sodium you lost from sweating by consuming sports drinks like Gatorade.

10. **Bring small energy boosts with you during your longer (30-minute) Steady Runs and workouts.** A very small snack or treat can be an excellent way to perk up when you're near the point of wanting to quit a harder effort. Some examples of energy boosts are: a handful of gummy bears, trail mix, or one or two packets of honey. Note that these are very small quantities and the minimal amount of glycogen in them should help give you a quick shot of energy to get you through a rough patch of training.

Symptoms of Overtraining

Everyone responds to training differently. Each individual approaches these schedules with their own existing level of fitness, weight, and attitude. If you've got a good case of the running "bug" after reading this book then you might dive right into training. You'll try to do everything I've suggested and, perhaps, at some point you may have dove too deep into the sport. I want you to fall in love with running for the rest of your life, and so I owe you a few paragraphs about how to avoid going too hard and overtraining. If you are experiencing any of these symptoms, then you may be running too hard and too much. In that case, take a few "rest and recover" days regardless of what the schedule tells you to do. Listening to your body when it's overtrained is paramount. Overtraining can lead to burnout, and burnout can lead to quitting the sport altogether. It can also be a great way to get injured.

- **You're having trouble sleeping.** One of the reasons I've asked you to annotate your sleeping patterns in your training log is that the body sometimes can rebel against the thing it needs most. Excessive running or running too hard can lead to insomnia. If you are experiencing bouts of sleeplessness after several hard workouts, then it's time to dial back.

- **You're feeling "fried."** You dread doing all your workouts. You have no energy—totally burned out. Overtraining can cause mental fatigue along with physical fatigue. If you just can't bring yourself to the track or up the hill for a harder workout, then cut yourself a break and regroup. Perhaps use one of your "attaboy/attagirl" rewards you've saved up to boost your morale.

- **Your loved ones are telling you that you're being unusually grouchy.** Working too hard can lead to irritability. Pay attention to what people say about your mood. Check your training log to see if there's a correlation with your training, and reduce your running if need be.

Preparing for the Niggles

If you have never run before, you probably don't know what to expect in terms of aches and pains. Something that may seem like the end of your brief running career could be a small "niggle." On the other hand, you may think that you should gut through a deep pain in your knee when, in fact, it's something that requires immediate medical attention. So what is acceptable and what isn't?

First off, defer to the guidance of a physician above all else when you're experiencing pain. Ultimately, doctors know best.

Here are symptoms that should serve as warning signs that you should probably rest and consider seeking medical care:

- **Acute, sharp, sudden pain in any part of your body.** If it's enough to make you wince, limp, or cry out, then unfortunately you are probably dealing with something serious.
- **Persistent swelling of a particular area.** Swelling usually means immediate rest and a doctor's visit.
- **Excessive breathing problems when trying to run.** When in doubt as to whether or not anything tied to your heart rate or breathing is normal, seek advice from your doctor.

Running in the Elements

To be a successful runner, you have to become a bit of an amateur meteorologist. In the next few months you may be spending more time than you ever have outside. As such, you should know as much as possible about the conditions you will eventually face. Every week, check out your forecast and annotate the following data points in your log: daily high and low temperatures, if rain or snow are expected, the wind speed and direction, as well as the dew point.

Note that if you are doing a "hard" workout like speed work, you will certainly struggle more in weather conditions that are less than ideal. Be prepared to run your "hard" lap at a slower pace than you ran it on days in better weather.

The Dew Point

This piece of meteorological data is often overlooked, which is unfortunate, because I consider it to be the best gauge for how uncomfortable you will feel in terms of humidity. Simply put, the dew point is a measure of how much moisture is in the air. The higher the dew point, the more "balmy" you will feel. If you live in Florida, you can experience days where the dew point is over 70 degrees Fahrenheit. Anything in the high 60s will make your runs that much more challenging. You have to be very careful when running during these high dew point days. Carry extra water with you and take frequent walk breaks on your longer Steady Runs. During these breaks pour some water over your head to cooldown. Don't forget to load up with electrolyte-heavy sports drinks after your run to replace all the salts that you sweat out.

The Wind

If you've never run before and think about heading outdoors, then you probably are most concerned about the temperature. This is a valid thing to worry about, but one factor often forgotten by beginners is the wind. A walk or a run on a long stretch of flat road into a driving headwind can be brutal. If you are attempting something like this on an "easy" day, then you may be setting yourself up for failure. By doing the right planning using your training log, you should be aware of what the expected wind will be like. If you are to experience blustery head-winds, then consider changing your route or even switching out your workout for a day when the winds are calmer. Also, think about finding one or two of your staple run routes that are more protected from the winds.

The Sun

A difficult workout will be that much harder if you have to squint or are stuck with the sun in your face the entire time. When you are running in uncomfortable zones of pain and exhaustion, a pair of sunglasses and a light hat with a brim can help.

The Cold

If you look at the starting line of a large race on a cold day, you can quickly see those who know how to run in the cold and those who don't. One of the biggest mistakes that novice runners make in the winter is overdressing. They look outside the window, check the thermometer, and then stick their nose out into the cold, only to decide to layer up with way too much clothing. They do this because even though they are getting prepared to run, their body has been at a state of rest. The difference with running is that you will be generating a lot of heat and so you don't need to wear a thick coat and lined sweats. A good rule of thumb is that they want to feel moderately chilly before they depart on their run. If they feel warm before even taking a step down the road, then they are overdressed. Overdressing can cause a lot of problems. It can increase your sweat rate, which can lead to dehydration, and it can simply be a big inconvenience—when you feel too hot, it increases the chances that you'll want to quit your run or cut back on it. Knowing exactly how much to wear or not wear takes years of practice. Your best way to get it right is to wear many layers of long-sleeved shirts. As you start out your run, you will perhaps feel cold, but once you've hit your groove, you will start to feel too warm. At that point you can shed one of your thin layers. Thin, long-sleeved shirts can be rolled up and stuffed into your pockets or even tied around your waist.

Another temperature toggle that you have at your disposal is your head, which gives off a lot of heat. Wear a knit cap on days when the temps dip below freezing and if you start to get too hot, take it off. If you find yourself running on a day where the wind chill is a factor, then make sure you've got on a wind-resistant jacket over those thin layers of long-sleeved shirts. Another thing I like to do when it's cold out is wear a pair of cheap cotton gloves that I bought for a buck at a dollar store. I even keep an extra pair of them in pocket in the event that I need to wipe my nose or brow or get my hands wet and require a replacement pair. Lastly, don't forget that when you're done with your run, you are going to start getting cold FAST. Your body stops generating heat and worse, you're all wet from sweat. Get indoors after your winter runs and either hop in the shower or quickly change into a comfy pair of dry, warm sweats that you've kept near your radiator or heating vent while you've been outside on the roads.

The Ice and Snow

A patch of black ice is probably the worst thing a runner can encounter out on the roads. A quick, unexpected slip and all that hard work could be lost with a broken bone. As such, I strongly recommend that you not run at all outside during icy conditions. Head to a vacant parking garage or a suburban mall instead. If it's snowing out, use your judgement, because snow and ice usually go together. Run a block or two to test the conditions first. Snow running can be a lot of fun, but be aware that any run in the snow should be considered a "hard" workout. Your stride has to change due to the unique running surface, and the softness of the snow prevents you from being able to run fast. If you get a lot of snow (three or more inches), then consider doing a deep snow walk as an alternate to whatever you have on your schedule.

The Night

Running in low-light conditions—the evening or the early morning— can feel incredibly liberating. Many people aren't out and about and so oftentimes if feels like it's just you and the road. But you have to take necessary precautions for these challenging conditions. Wear reflective clothing and consider buying a few of those clip-on LED lights that you can attach to parts of your body. It's much easier to trip or fall when you can't see so well, which means you should slow down your pace on any low-light runs. Also make sure that you've done some good route research. Before you run on a stretch of road at night, perhaps consider driving it to see what the lighting conditions are. Stay off dark, unlit country roads. It's also possible to experience sudden night blindness when your eyes have to deal with the glare of a car's oncoming headlights. One technique to preserve your night vision when this happens is to close one eye and keep one eye open. Open your closed eye after that blinding car has passed you. Take extra precautions with your gear during your low-light runs. Consider packing a small flashlight. If you run with a smartphone, ensure that it has a full charge in the event you need to call for help. Finally, it can be dangerous out there on the roads at night, so find a running buddy that can accompany you on these types of runs.

Warming Up

Before you do any exercise or workout prescribed in this book, you need to get yourself ready. No matter the workout, it's imperative that you warm up the body a bit. A sudden jolt to the system can increase the chances of injury, so make sure you transition to your workout properly. The warmup that I want you to be doing doesn't have to take a long time and doesn't need to be over-analyzed. All I want you to do for a warmup is spend two to three minutes doing something easy that puts your body in motion. It can be a slow walk for that period of time before you head into a run, or it can be something like a 10 to 15 jumping jacks or jogging in place for 30 seconds at a time. The aim here is to get your heart rate up a bit and your body in motion. The only exception to this warmup routine is when you are doing lap repeats on your speed work days. Recall that those specifics are explained in the speed work section of this chapter (see page 32).

Cooling Down

Just as the body needs to warm up before a run, so too does it need to transition into a cooldown. Your cooldown can be the same thing as your warmup—two to three minutes of slow movement—preferably a nice and slow walk. End your workout with a positive affirmation. Reflect on what went well during the run and don't forget to jot down your feelings about the workout in your training log.

To Stretch or Not to Stretch . . .

Many running books dedicate entire chapters to stretching. All you will get from me is a paragraph and no specific stretches that I want you to try. I'm not a big fan of stretching—especially before a run when the body isn't warmed up. I believe that prestretching muscle fibers that have not had much blood warming them up is similar to trying to immediately start a car in the cold and taking it at 100 miles per hour. The best way for muscles to warm up is to get them in motion through walking or slow running and not by stretching them unnecessarily. This advice is based on twenty-five years of personal experience and coaching. If you feel stretching helps you, then do it after your run at the end of your cooldown period. Here are a few dos and don'ts with regards to stretching:

- **Do:** stay in your comfort zone with your stretches. You shouldn't be in any pain at all while you stretch.
- **Don't:** hold your breath while holding your stretches.
- **Don't:** "bounce" or rock your body back and forth in order to touch or reach a further point on your body.

Dealing with Technology

My first training book, *Run Simple,* was about how to liberate yourself from running technology and learn how to listen to your body. So, not surprisingly, I'm not a proponent of overreliance on GPS and heart rate monitors. I'm also not a big fan of listening to music on the run, because I think it prevents a true mind/body connection and can be dangerous in traffic. Experiment with simplicity. Our lives are complicated and busy enough already outside of running. Try to use your 30 minutes a day as a peaceful time to take a break from the smartphone notifications that constantly bombard us. Instead of listening to music, experience the world around you in its natural state. Do your workout in a nature preserve and listen to the birds. Your mind will crave this daily shot of tranquil quality time.

Another piece of technology that you should be careful of is the Internet. In just a few minutes on Google, you can find a horde of conflicting information about various running topics. Be careful with relying on this information for advice. Running "trolls" abound out there, stalking online running forums. It's better to get your running support by joining a local club than from a bunch of people you've never met dwelling on the Internet.

But there is one element of technology that you can benefit from: the healthy use of social media. A close group of family or friends on Facebook can be a huge support to you as you start your new routine. Posting your achievements for them to "like" is a great way to gain emotional support. Consider also giving the "likes" back to your fellow runners who are out to achieve their own goals.

Conducting a "System Check"

Complex machinery like a car or an airplane operate successfully thanks to gauges. These serve as a way for the pilot or driver to monitor what is happening while the machine is in operation. Gauges can serve as warning signs that assist with problem solving. When you start out on a training run, I would like you to monitor your body's own "gauges" so that you can take appropriate actions to ensure you avoid injury and make the most of your workout. Starting from the bottom and ending at the top, here are the moving pieces and parts that you need to monitor. Ask yourself the following questions when you are doing your own "system" check. You should do this check during the first five minutes, at the mid-point, and near the end of your run.

Your feet. How does each stride feel? Are your toes comfortable? Do your laces seem too loose or tight? Any rocks or wood chips in your shoes? If, after the first minute of your run you sense anything is wrong with your feet, then stop and take action like loosening your laces or emptying that annoying rock. Any problem like this that is not addressed right away will only get worse the longer you run. You risk developing a blister or a hot spot that could only lead to more trouble so stopping to get your feet comfortable is much more important than "suffering" through a run because you don't want to stop or feel that you will not get the right cardiovascular stimulus.

Your knees. A bit of the popping at the beginning of a run, especially in the cold, is normal for older runners. But if you experience pain from the onset that continues to worsen throughout the run, then it could be your IT band or something worse, and so you probably should stop the run and return home. Ice and elevate your problem knee and consider taking a day off or doing some cross-training like swimming until it feels better.

Your legs. How do your calves feel? How about your thighs? If you've got some dull aches and pains, especially if you did some faster running or accomplished a milestone like running for 30 minutes without stopping earlier in the training week, this may be cause for the soreness. If you were doing speed work, then you may feel it in your calves, because faster running usually means running on the balls of our feet, which stresses the calf muscle. Try to know what to expect if you feel any of these pains and learn about your body by seeking to understand the causes for anything that feels out of the ordinary.

Your torso. Is there any cramping going on? Do you feel a side stitch? If so, then stop running and walk for at least five minutes before resuming your run. Why do you think you are cramping? Do you think you ate a meal too soon after your workout? Or perhaps you downed a bottle of water too fast? Again, question the pains you feel and try to get to the root of the problem so that you can prevent it from happening again. Another reason for any kind of torso (abdominal or back) pain might be related to cross-training exercises you completed in the training week. The stronger your "core" becomes, the less pain you should feel when running.

Your lungs. How heavy are you breathing? Unless you are doing some speed-work laps, you should be breathing comfortably and able to have a short conversation with a training partner. Any pained breathing is probably a warning sign. What does your breathing sound like? Close one ear and listen to your lungs at work. Are you wheezing? If your breathing is erratic, then slow it down or stop altogether.

Your arms. How are you carrying your arms? Are they swinging excessively high or not enough? Are you swinging your arms in one direction or are they swinging at an angle? What do your hands feel like? Are you clenching your fists? Unless you are running up a hill, everything dealing with your arms should be relaxed and normal. You shouldn't feel tight anywhere. Your hands should feel comfortable—no squeezing. The fingers shouldn't be touching each other. If they are, you may be feeling a dull pain creeping up your arms to your neck and shoulders.

Your head, neck, and shoulders. Is your neck stiff? Do you have any shoulder pain? If so, this may stem from how you are carrying your arms and if you are clenching your hands. Relax! Tension in the body tends to accumulate in this area. How does your head feel? I don't mean your hair; I mean your mind. This is the most important gauge that you can monitor. Is your head in the game? Are you motivated? Do you have any doubts or fears about your run? Are you bored? If your mind is restless and troubled, then tell yourself positive affirmations. For example, if you are stressed that you might not be able to make through without quitting, then visualize the last successful workout you completed. If you're bored, think about something fun that you have planned later that day or week. Try to nip the "stinking running" thinking in the bud. Negative thoughts can quickly get out of control. If you can't seem to shake them, it's OK to do a few walk/runs to compose yourself. Another technique you can employ if you sense that you are struggling with the mental aspects of your run is distraction. Fixate on landmarks along your route, focus on some nonrunning aspect of your life such as your work, or perhaps take a mental inventory of your kitchen and plan your next grocery trip. If it's the holiday season, come up with your gift list. Anything other than thinking about the moment you're in along the run could be what you need to tide you over a bad mental patch.

What to Do after You Take Off Your Running Shoes

Once you've completed your workout, there are some important things you need to do to ensure that you will be able to prepare for your next workout. Earlier in this chapter, I covered the importance of recovery nutrition and hydration.

- **Drink.** Immediately rehydrate with a few glasses of water as well as one sports drink (or a glass of chocolate milk).

- **Stretch.** If you feel up to it, do some light stretching but nothing that causes any pain.
- **Eat.** An hour after your workout, have a light snack like a whole wheat bagel or a banana.
- **Put your feet up.** Your body has been in a vertical position for a long period of time. Your heart has to work especially hard to push blood down to the bottoms of your toes; therefore, a good idea is to elevate your feet as a way to ensure optimal blood flow to all those tendons, capillaries, and ligaments.
- **Do a "mirror check."** As you start to undergo your equilibrium shift, you will begin to notice small, positive changes to your body. Your pants will start to feel less tight. Your neck, wrists, and stomach will thin. Your legs will feel lean and strong. These are all incredible changes that you deserve to discover. Get in the habit of looking at yourself in a full-length mirror, and tell yourself that all this hard work is starting to really pay off.
- **Go to bed early.** Your body needs the rest.

Safety

If you're new to running then you've got to understand that training out on the roads or trails in difficult conditions can mean that you will, sooner or later, encounter some unsafe events. I like to think of these instead as "adventures," but the good news is that most of the things that can go wrong out in the elements are preventable. Here are some safety basics that you should follow to ensure your runs don't turn into near-death experiences:

- **Don't run with traffic; run against it.** This may seem counterintuitive, but running against traffic allows you to see any potential threats, like a distracted driver, and react accordingly. If you run with traffic, you won't be able to hear or see the possible threats.

- **Make eye contact with drivers.** It seems like more and more drivers these days are staring at the electronic screens and not the roads. Once you make eye contact with a driver, you can almost always tell if they are paying attention or not. If they aren't, then run off the road and stop until they pass.

- **Be aware of sun blindness.** A well-behaved driver may be paying attention to the road and still not see you if it's the evening or morning and they are blinded by a setting/rising sun. A good way to notice that this phenomenon is occurring is to look at the visors of the cars that pass you. Are they down with the drivers peering under them? If so, consider changing your route. To avoid this problem altogether, then avoid running at sunrise or sunset.

- **Give yourself exits.** When I'm running, I am constantly scanning in front of me for any vehicular threats. I'm also planning how I can exit the road if a driver doesn't see me. Try to avoid routes that don't have any exits for you. The wider the shoulder, the better.

- **Don't listen to music while you run.** Music in your ears prevents you from hearing traffic around you. If you feel that music helps you, then just use one earphone and keep one ear listening to your surroundings.

- **Wear reflective clothing.** Buy running clothes that come with reflective material sewn on it. If you don't want to invest in these, then you can order cheaper reflective fabric and safety-pin or sew that onto your clothes. You can also purchase little clip-on LED flashing lights. Another option is to purchase a headlamp to run with, but for beginners, these can be yet another piece of equipment that can cause frustration (and require batteries).

- **Don't run in dark places at night.** If you are going to be doing darkness or low-light runs, then find routes with ample streetlights.

- **Use the buddy system.** Not only are running buddies great to help you push yourself when you want to quit, but they also can give you peace of mind about safety in the event something goes wrong out on the roads or trails.

- **Tell people where you are going and how long you will be gone.** As a courtesy to your loved ones, especially if you are going to be out for a longer workout or at night, make sure you let them know where you are going on your run and what route you are taking. Another option is to give your loved ones a list of your typical routes so that they know where you are.

- **Bring ID with you as well as info as to medicines you take and your blood type.** You never know what can happen on a run, and it's good to prepare in the event that medical professionals need to care for you if you are unable to communicate.

- **Stick a few dollars in your sock or threaded between your laces.** It's good to have a bit of cash on you in the event you need to stop in a convenience store to grab an essential drink or snack.

- **Know where you can get free water along the way.** The last thing you want to have to worry about on your run is being thirsty. Do some planning in advance and know a few places along your route where you can get free water. Most convenience stores or restaurants will give a thirsty runner a glass of free water. And many city parks have public water fountains. Do the same planning for public restrooms as well.

Running on Trails

Not all your training runs need to take place on the roads and tracks. In fact, constant running on harder surfaces like asphalt can increase the chances of injury to your legs. As you start to plan out your running routes, consider doing at least one workout on the trails. But before you wander out into a state park or forest preserve, take into account these four differences in trail versus road running:

1. **Trails provide more demanding workouts.** Even though the dirt and grass can offer you a welcome break from the intensity of the roads, they are usually harder to run on. Many single-track trails present challenges like winding twists and turns, root structures, and rocks. These obstacles mean that you will be bounding and leaping vertically in ways that you aren't used to on the roads. So if this is your first trail run, take it easy. Consider walk/running the first time you run on a trail and be sure to stop a run to step over an obstacle. Trails also provide more of a mental challenge. It's harder to "zone out" on a trail run, as you need to be constantly paying attention to the trail before you. Because of this increased difficulty, don't do any speed work or steady runs on the trails. Instead use the trails as a place to do your walk and walk/run workouts.

2. **Trails can be less safe than roads.** You won't have to worry about distracted drivers out on the trails, but you do have to worry about the consequences of getting lost or injured while out in nature. As such, run your first few trail workouts with a buddy. Bring along a mobile phone, as well as extra water and snacks in the event your workout lasts longer than expected. Plan your route in advance and if you are running on the trails alone, let a loved one know where on the trails you are planning

to go and when you are expecting to return. Learn about the trail network. Read about it on the Web. Ask yourself questions like: Are there water fountains or restrooms? How hilly is the route? What will conditions be like on the day of the run? Are the trails possibly washed out or excessively muddy? If you've never run on a particular trail, then plan on doing your first few workouts as "out and back," where you run out along the trail for half of your prescribed time and then turn around and run back. This will help prevent you from getting lost or accidentally making a wrong turn if you are fatigued.

3. **Trails are good places for gear.** You don't have to get fancy, but it might be a good idea to purchase a small running pouch that you can attach around your waist. In this pouch, carry energy bars, Vaseline (for chafing), Band-Aids, moleskin, your car keys, and even bug repellant. Consider also buying a water bottle that fits around your hand. One thing you don't need to buy, however, are special trail-running shoes. The duration and frequency of your trail workouts don't require this added purchase. Your regular running shoes should suffice.

4. **Trails aren't for electronics.** Besides the benefits of leaping and bounding over obstacles, trails also can be the perfect places to mentally "unplug." Many trail networks don't get good GPS satellite reception, so don't try to use the trails to measure your pace or distance. Run simple. Don't wear headphones; listen to the birds instead and commune with nature.

Grass and Sand

Occasionally, switching up the actual surface that you run on can change the stimulation of the run itself. If your feet are feeling tired after a difficult workout, think about switching the surface you run on in your next workout to short grass. Find a large, soft, dry area like a golf course or a stretch of field in a park and run there. Grass is an excellent natural cushion and far preferable to running on asphalt. Seek out these areas as locations to give yourself a break. Along the same lines, the beach may also seem like an optimal place in order to run a relaxing workout, but be careful. The "give" of a soft, sandy surface can act like a resistance workout, similar to running in the snow. And if you are running on hard, wet sand, it can also have a similar effect to running on pavement. Beaches seem like wonderful locales for running, but I would caution you to avoid them if you are a first-time runner. They typically don't have any shade, and combined with the rigors of running on sand, they are best left for you to vacation at. Skip the beach, and find the grass.

Putting It All Together

This is the longest chapter in the book, and if the concept of running is new to you, then you might be feeling a bit overwhelmed by all this advice and direction. Let me try to help assuage your concerns by writing out a narrative that weaves together most of the elements of training I've written about here. I will use the following two-week sample for demonstrative purposes.

Sample Week 1: Your purpose this week is to complete "Base Building." The week's example schedule looks like this:

Mon	Tues	Wed	Thurs	Fri	Sat	Sun
Easy, Walk, 20	Rest	Medium, Run/ Walk, 25 (3/2)	Rest	Easy, Walk, 20	Rest	Easy, Walk, 15

This week should be annotated in your training log. The weekend before this week, you sit down and study the plan. You look at the forecasted weather and write down the temperatures (high/low), wind speed, and direction. You also cross-reference the plan with your work schedule. You ask yourself if this plan is doable given the conditions and your personal schedule. It is, but you notice that the temperatures will be below freezing in the morning on the Wednesday that you are supposed to do your medium run/walk of 30 minutes, so you plan to do your workout at lunch when the temperatures are highest and you won't have to worry about the dangers of black ice.

On Monday, you wake up early for your 20-minute walk. You have a light breakfast of toast and honey with a cup of coffee. You down a tall glass of water. Two hours later, you put on your workout clothes and head out for your walk. You pick a new route for this particular walk, because you want to explore a small trail network in a nearby park. You feel great and discover a lot of other trail options you can take on your next walk. When you get back home, you do some light stretching. You drink a tall glass of chocolate milk and eat a banana with a handful of peanuts. Your left calf is a little sore a few hours after your walk. You elevate your feet and unwind by watching your favorite show with a bag of frozen peas wrapped around your left leg. You usually go to bed at 10pm, but decide to get some extra sleep and hit the sack at 9pm.

On Tuesday, you take the day off. You go grocery shopping and remember that you are trying to stay on the "edges" of the store. You suddenly realize that you are in the junk food aisle and with your favorite snack in your shopping cart: chocolate chip cookies. You put them back and substitute with a bag of apples on the left wall of the store. You remember that you need to shift your equilibrium and that making changes means encountering resistance and applying discipline like this to affect positive change. When you are done with dinner you decide to look at your workout for tomorrow and notice that the forecast is now calling for two inches of snow. You decide that your run/walk workout might be treacherous outside, so instead, you switch this workout with Friday's easy 20-minute walk, because the snow is supposed to melt by that point. So you make the following changes to your weekly schedule:

Mon	Tues	Wed	Thurs	Fri	Sat	Sun
Easy, Walk, 20	Rest	~~Medium, run/walk, (3/2), 25~~ Easy, Walk, 20	Rest	~~Easy, Walk, 20~~ Medium, Run/Walk, 25 (3/2)	Rest	Easy, Walk, 15

On Wednesday, you wake up and look outside. The snow has started. It's supposed to taper off by noon, so you choose to do your 15-minute walk then. You dress in three layers of long-sleeved shirts, running tights, a knit cap, and gloves. You are a bit on the chilly side, but you know that once you start walking, your body will generate the extra heat to make you feel comfortable. You know that it's harder to walk in the snow, so you choose a route with wide sidewalks in the city that are plowed. Your legs feel great at first, but eight minutes into the walk, you start to really hurt. The snow was deeper in parts than you realized, and you are getting tired. You make the call to cut your walk short by five minutes, because you know that walking or running in the snow is much more difficult than in clear conditions.

You get Thursday off and try out a new recipe using whole-wheat pasta. You realize you forgot to update your running journal for the week, so you spend a few minutes before bed logging your training. You write about the nice new trails you found on Monday and about the fact that you had some soreness in your left calf that day, but it doesn't hurt anymore. Right before bedtime, you decide to do some meditation. You go into a spare room in your house and draw the curtains. You sit down on a mat on the floor, light a candle, and relax. You visualize tomorrow's workout and make some positive affirmations about how you will feel during it as you inhale. You exhale all negative emotions, imagining the positive replacing the negative. You get to bed before 10pm.

On Friday, you are to do a medium-effort workout of 25 minutes where you walk three minutes and then run two minutes for the duration of that time period. The temperatures are above freezing and that day's high is supposed to be in the 50s, but the winds are expected to be blustery. You have a light snack (an apple and a handful of macadamia nuts) at 10 am and decide to do your workout at 11:30. The winds are picking up once you start your workout. After the fifth minute of your walk, you start to run. It's only the second time you've tried a run longer than a minute and so you're not confident that you can make it. You feel the wind in your face and each step seems to get increasingly harder. But you take a quick "system check" and all your "gauges" seem to be holding up. One minute passes, then, two, then three. You did it! You walk for another three minutes and when it's time to start your next three-minute run, you are confident that you can make it. The rest of your workout is a success. You cooldown with a two-minute walk around your block. You down a glass of Gatorade and eat a whole wheat bagel with peanut butter on it. You change out of your wet and cold clothes and take a shower. Your legs really ache so you elevate them, putting bags of frozen peas on the areas that bother you most. You write about your success in your journal.

Saturday is a day off. You go through your kitchen and get rid of all junk food.

Sunday you walk for 15 minutes around your town, and that night you look ahead at your schedule for the second week, writing out the forecasted conditions like you did the week before. Your second week looks like this:

Sample Week 2: Your purpose this week is to do speed work.

Mon	Tues	Wed	Thurs	Fri	Sat	Sun

Rest	Rest	Hard, Speed Work
		• 5-minute warmup
		• 1 Steady lap
		• 3 Hard laps with
		  2 minute Rest
		  between
		• 5-minute Cooldown
			Rest	Easy, Walk,
				20
					Rest	Hard, Speed Work
						• 5-minute warmup
						• 1 Steady lap
						• 3 Hard laps with
						  2-minute Rest
						  between
						• 5-minute Cooldown

This is going to be a tough week for you. You will be running at speeds a little outside your comfort zone, but your success the week before has you confident that you will try. You remember the three training maxims—especially #1, that doing something is better than nothing. The weather looks good for the week, so you plan to do all your workouts in the morning. You get two rest days right at the start so that you can be ready for the speed work you will have to do on Wednesday. On Monday you feel great, so you decide to go for a swim at your friend's gym. You aren't a strong swimmer, so you decide to walk laps in a warm pool for 20 minutes. When you get home from your swim, you drink two glasses of water, but notice that the color of your urine is dark yellow so you drink another glass of water as well as a small Gatorade and have a few handfuls of trail mix with a hard-boiled egg.

Tuesday, you don't do any exercise but meditate in the morning. At night, you start to think about the workout ahead of you. You are worried about how the fast laps will feel and you aren't sure if you will be able to run at the correct pace. You're also concerned that you may get injured by running so fast. You journal all these thoughts in your log, and it makes you feel better that you got it out.

Then it is Wednesday. Luckily, you live about five minutes' walk away from the track, so you use that as your warmup. When you get to the track, you walk one lap around it to familiarize your mind and body with what to expect and then put the water bottle and two energy bars you brought with you in the stands near the start. You reset your watch and run one "steady" lap around the track. Since this is a steady lap, you make sure you aren't running it too fast. You notice that the first half of the 400m, you start to feel like you are breathing too hard and so you slow it down almost to a walk. You hit the stop button on your watch and go over to the bleachers where your things are and write that time in your log that you brought with you. You take five minutes to compose yourself and then do your first hard lap. By the first 200m, you realize that you have gone out at a full sprint and that you are not going to be able to keep this up. You can barely breathe and your legs can't seem to move any faster. You slow down almost to the "steady" pace. When you come to the finish you realize you ran that lap eight seconds faster than your steady lap, so you are pleased. You walk over to your log and write this time down. You take a small gulp of water. The workout indicates that you are to do a 2-minute rest period, so you walk around the track for one minute and then walk across the infield to the start for the second minute. You run your second hard lap at a better sustained pace and do that one six seconds faster than your "steady" lap. You do the same 2-minute walk around the track, and then do your final lap. This one really hurts, and you are able to do it only one second faster than your "steady" lap. You write this time in your log, and then do a 5-minute walk home. You eat your energy bars and drink the rest of your water on your walk home. You stretch, elevate, and ice. At night, you study your log and realize that you probably went out too fast in your first lap and will remember that for your workout on Sunday.

You follow the schedule for Thursday, Friday, and Saturday and update your log.

It is finally Sunday. You complete the same workout and notice that each of your hard laps was five to six seconds faster than your steady lap. You then notice that your steady lap was three seconds faster than it was Wednesday. You realize that you have made significant improvements in your speed in just a few days' time. When you get back home, you post these impressive results on Facebook and tell your friends in your running network about your success. You realize that all this hard work, diligent planning, and discipline for the past two weeks hasn't been easy, but it has paid off. You are starting to make the equilibrium shift!

Sample Training Week 3 looks like this:

Sample Week 3: Your purpose this week is to do Speed Work/Hills.

Mon	Tues	Wed	Thurs	Fri	Sat	Sun
Rest	Cross-Training • Plank 3 × 30 secs • 10 Burpees • Standing Bicycle Crunches 2 × 20	Easy, Walk, 30	Rest	Hard, Hills • 15-minute Walk • 3 Hills • 5-minute Cooldown	Rest	Hard, Hills • 15-minute Walk • 4 Hills • 5-minute Cooldown

For illustrative purposes, I would like to focus just on your Tuesday and Friday workouts, since cross-training and hills haven't been covered yet in this example. As you prepare for your training week, you look ahead and see that you will be doing two hard workouts near the end of it. You've never done a hill workout, so you decide that on your rest day of Monday you will take a walk to look at two hills down the road from your house that might be good candidates on which to complete your workout. The first hill is really steep and long. You measure it with a GPS and find that it's about 700 feet in length. The other hill is less steep and much shorter. You measure it to be 400 feet. You decide you will try that one on Friday. On Tuesday, you take a short 10-minute walk around your neighborhood and then decide to do your three cross-training exercises for the day. Your first exercise is the Plank, and you head to your spare room and roll out your exercise mat. You get into the push-up position and then rest your forearms on the ground and put your toes up on the balls of your feet. You set your timer for 30 seconds and begin, but after a few seconds, you find that you are holding your breath and can't hold your back up. You drop to the floor. You don't get discouraged and remember that this is the first time you are attempting this exercise. You put your knees on the ground and set your watch for 30 seconds. You remember to breathe through the exercise. Thirty seconds passes and you stand up and shake out your legs. When you feel comfortable and ready, you do another two sets of the same exercise. You feel thirsty, and so you grab a drink of Gatorade that you brought with you into your exercise room. Your next exercise is the Burpee. You are supposed to do 10 reps, but can only do six. You take a break and stretch your arms and legs. You do the next four reps and remember to make sure that you are doing them slowly and methodically. You realize you were rushing too fast through the first six and getting too sloppy. You stand up, stretch out your arms and decide to take a break for a few minutes. You check your work email and then come back after 10 minutes to do your last exercise routine: the Standing Bicycle Crunch. You do two of these and lose your balance immediately. You remember that you can use a wall for support so you walk over to the side of your exercise room and do 20 reps. You take a minute break between the sets and finish up the last 20 reps with no problem. On Friday, you do your 15-minute walk using a route that gets you to the nearby hill that you selected on your Monday reconnaissance. You take a few minutes to shake out your legs and then run up the hill for your first repetition. You've never run up a hill like this before in your life and it really hurts. You feel like you are going too fast and so you slow down so that you can breathe easier. When you crest the hill, you transition to a walk, turn around, and walk back down the hill. As soon as you get to the base of the hill, you turn around and run back up it—remembering to pump your arms. It feels easier this time because you didn't go out so fast. On your third repetition, your legs are burning and you are completely out of breath. You walk back down the hill and return to your house to cool down your legs. Your glass of chocolate milk awaits you in the fridge, and you decide to do some very light stretching of your quadriceps. That next day, your legs are incredibly sore, and you decide to take a 5-minute walk around the block to get your heart moving so that it can help flush that lactic acid you have accumulated from your workout. Sunday's hill workout is very difficult. You don't think that one day was enough rest, but you are committed to try the workout. The first three hill repeats are incredibly challenging. You want to quit the workout, but remember that you have to put in the work to make the equilibrium shift, and so you do a fourth rep. Halfway up the hill you stop running and walk to the top. You remember Training Maxim #1 (doing something is better than nothing), so you walk back down the hill and do your last repeat by running as much as you can. You run about 100 feet and then walk again, but you crest the hill and return home exhausted. You are proud of yourself that you did the workout even though it wasn't easy. You write down what you learned about yourself in your training log and reward yourself with a dinner out to your favorite Italian restaurant with your spouse.

Frequently Asked Questions

If you've made it this far into the book, then you might be questioning a few key concepts—how to apply the principles I've outlined in this chapter. What follows are some answers to the common questions that my beginner athletes ask me about their training:

Can I make changes to the schedules? If so, how? Absolutely. As I've indicated earlier, it's imperative that you approach your 30-minute training with an open mind. These schedules are merely guideposts for you. Feel free to substitute training days within the week, but never complete back-to-back "hard" effort days. Err on the side of caution and if you have to skip one workout a week, that's OK.

I'm worried that I may be too heavy to start running. What can I do?

During your first run/walk, if you can't run for the minimum time (one minute), then simply substitute that run period with a walk. Replace all running in the schedule with walking and believe in yourself. Walking, combined with good nutrition, should lead to weight loss, and these pounds you are able to shed thanks to walking will make running that much easier. Most 5K races don't restrict you from walking the entire distance, so, though this is mostly a book about running, there is nothing wrong with completing a 5K race without ever breaking your stride. Eventually, you should be able to walk/run. After you've been able to complete a 5K by walking, follow one of these training schedules and give running a shot.

I don't have a track near where I live. How do I do the speed work?
You don't have to have a track to do your speed work. Find a flat stretch of road or trail and measure out approximately 1,200 feet. Do your "laps" there. Tracks are great to run on because of their softer surface and their oval shape, but aren't mandatory to your training.

I don't have a hill near where I live. How do I do the hills?
If you have any sort of hill—even one with a small grade—that's fine. If you have no options then make the hill workout a "steady" run instead.

I've started the schedule and I'm not making any progress. What can I do? Don't give up. If you are advancing in the schedule and are encountering more challenging workouts that you are unable to achieve, then repeat a week until you are able to complete all those workouts. If you're feeling mentally and physically burned out, then read about some motivational strategies in the next chapter.

Do I have to jog when I am resting between laps on my speed work days? No. It's perfectly OK to walk during this period. Staying moving is important, so don't sit or lie down. If you feel compelled to do that then you are probably running your hard lap too fast and should back off. The goal of each fast lap isn't to run to the point of collapse, but to run at a slightly to moderately faster pace than your "steady" lap.

Is there ever a day where it will be too hot or cold to run?
Safety first. If the temperatures, winds, or dew point are at intolerable levels, then don't do the workout that day. You can substitute a cross-training day in the place of a run or you can head to a large indoor space like a shopping mall or an empty parking garage where you can do your workouts in a more favorable setting. Hopefully you will have planned ahead by using your training log

and have shifted your schedule around to ensure you're doing the workouts on the best-possible day of the week.

I tried the first-time run schedule in this book, and I think I need a coach. Is that OK? If so, how should I find the right coach for me?

I think that exercising for no more than 30 minutes a day is all you need to achieve the goal of running your first 5K. This book *should* be enough. However, I would never discourage you from finding a coach. A good coach can definitely help you—especially if you are overweight and have never run before in your life. If you do decide to hire a coach, then try to find someone who listens more than asserts. Tell them about your goals. Show them this book and explain what you are trying to achieve by using it. If you've never run before and consider yourself to be out of shape, then you may want to look for a coach who can fulfill two needs: dietary and running. A nutritionist who also runs is a good example of someone who might be the best fit for you. Interview your coach much like you are interviewing someone at work. Ask them about their coaching philosophy. Find out their own background with the sport. Have they ever been overweight or out of shape? When did they first take up running? After listening to your background, how do they think they can complement the teachings espoused in this book? What is their fee schedule? Do they offer any rebate or refund if they aren't successful in assisting you? At a minimum, you should interview at least three coaches so that you can make an informed comparison. Some coaches offer virtual support (email/Skype/phone) while others who live near you can supervise you in person. The former is usually cheaper than the latter. If you've decided that you need a coach, then I recommend hiring someone you can meet in person at least for a few sessions so they can watch you run and get to know you better than just over the phone.

I want to run longer than 30 minutes. I don't think 30 minutes is long enough to work out. Is this OK?

The whole premise of this book is that 30 minutes max a day is more than enough time you need to work out to achieve your goals. But I don't want to discourage you from wanting to achieve more. If you've never run a 5K before and are doing either the first or second training schedule, then the short answer to your question is no. I want you to have completed at least one 5K before you venture out into workouts that last longer than 30 minutes. Chapter 6, Thrive, is all about how to take your running to this more advanced level.

How do I know when it's time to buy a new pair of running shoes? You indicated it's after 300 to 500 miles, but this book gives me my training in minutes instead.

Keep a running total of the cumulative minutes you compile in your log. Assuming you are averaging 10 minutes per mile, this means you should think about replacing your shoes at 10 x 300 or approximately 3,000 minutes of running (50 hours). When in doubt, go back to your shoe expert at your local running store and ask for their honest opinion after looking at the wear in the soles.

I can't do the Burpees cross-training exercise. It hurts too much to drop from a squat to the push-up position. Can I skip these?

Absolutely. If you are having a hard time doing these, then switch to the Plank with your knees on the ground. After a few weeks of training, look into experimenting with the Burpee again to see if it's easier. The goal for the duration of the schedule is to see if you can do one before you take part in your first 5K.

I can't run at all. How do I do the assigned speed work? Do your "steady" lap at a slow walk and do your hard laps at a fast, race-walk pace. You don't have to run these. You should just do them at a significantly faster pace than your "steady" lap.

I see a lot of people who like to run barefoot. Should I try that out? I strongly advise that you NOT dabble with barefoot running. There are many schools of thought about running "minimalism" and whether it's good for you or not. I sit strongly in the "do not run barefoot" camp. I don't subscribe to the theory that humans have evolved to run barefoot. I believe that excessive weight gain combined with a sedentary lifestyle in our modern world mean that we need cushioning on our feet in order to run. We also need stability. These elements, that are provided in the form of a nice pair of running shoes, will help ward off injury, so wear running shoes! Your knees and legs will thank you.

Should I put leg weights on or carry weights in my hands when I run? Absolutely not. Adding more weight to your body than what you are already used to carrying is a terrible idea and a recipe for a quick injury. Leave all weights at home; you don't need them.

You have advised against buying a running watch with GPS. Can I wear something similar, but less cumbersome, like a Fitbit? I'm OK with you using a basic Fitbit to supplement your training, but I would recommend relying more heavily on the simple, easy-to-comprehend workouts described in this book. However, if you want to use a Fitbit to help monitor your caloric intake and therefore lead you to making healthier nutritional choices and reducing your portion size, I think that could be beneficial. But that being said, it's much simpler to use this book as your guide, and there's no need to feel compelled to go out and buy technology to assist you. What you need to succeed you already have: a strong and committed mind that is capable of being disciplined, common sense, and a strong desire to change.

Chapter 4

CONQUER

This chapter is for the quitters.

I'm not joking. In fact, I want you to grab a bookmark and insert it here for the first time you feel like giving up on a run. Know that every runner—even a gold-medal Olympic marathoner—has at some point along their journey quit a workout. Therefore, if you want to run your first 5K, it's best to learn about when it's a good time to quit a workout and when it's best to keep going.

Running isn't easy, and there's something in the running culture that scorns people for quitting, which is a shame. Think of yourself as a mountain climber. Moving your body at a pace it's never reached before is very much like summiting the peak of a tall mountain.

All professional mountain climbers worth their salt know when they need to stop their summit attempt and simply climb back down to the bottom. A climber who refuses to quit in the face of treacherous conditions or lacking food and oxygen is a climber with a death wish. The risk rarely pays off. A good climber knows the mountain and is wise when it's just not the right time to push on.

I want you to accept the fact that as a new runner, sometimes it's OK to quit a workout. As much as it pains me to write this, I also feel compelled to tell you it's OK to quit running for a while if you become injured or burned out.

This chapter is also about motivation—how to use some simple mental tricks to stay in the game and not let the pesky forces of resistance prevent you from making your equilibrium shift. Finally, this chapter also covers how to run in unique circumstances—i.e., if you're a single parent learning how to incorporate your new hobby into your life or a person with a job that requires a lot of travel.

Let's take them one at a time and start with the concept of quitting.

When It's OK to Quit a Run

- **When you are experiencing acute pain—at any time.** Acute pain is a sharp pain that occurs when the body is sending up a red flag of distress. By all means, heed it and stop your running immediately. See a doctor if necessary and follow his/her advice.
- **When you are having trouble breathing.** Pained breathing is another red flag. Stop running immediately.
- **When you are training during a "Rest and Recover" week.** If you don't feel well, then write it off as a bad day and put your feet up and rest. Most likely your body is telling you that you should be resting anyway.

When It's Probably Not OK to Quit a Run

- **Unless you are feeling acute pain or are having excessive breathing problems, don't quit the first five minutes of any run.** Getting out the door is usually the hardest thing—especially if it's really cold out. The next-hardest thing is getting the body transitioning from a state of rest to a state of movement. Your body will tend to resist and rebel in the opening minutes. Your mind will make up excuses. Try to suffer through the beginning and realize that it can get easier as you start to warm up.
- **When you start to feel tired on a medium- or hard-intensity workout.** During these types of workouts, you have to push your body in order to strengthen it.
- **When you're too hot or cold.** If you've prepared properly, you can adjust your layers of clothing. Don't give in to the elements. Being over- or underdressed is not an excuse to quit.

Motivation

Sooner or later, you will encounter motivational issues. You'll look at your schedule and dread what's been prescribed for you. What follows are some coping strategies to deal with a case of the running "blahs."

- **Motivation Tip #1: Get a loved one to literally push you out the door.** No matter what. I've always told runners that I coach that simply getting out of the door is usually enough to fix any motivational issues. There seems to be some invisible force that forces us to stay indoors. This is especially true in the winter, when the body doesn't want to deal with the arctic air. When it's cold out, try to get your workout in during the warmest time of the day. Do the opposite during the summer.

- **Motivation Tip #2: Change your pace.** Sometimes the "blahs" set in when your body is bored with running. If you're walking and unmotivated, then do a 30-second run. The little shot of adrenaline may alter the tedious dynamic that caused the motivation problem in the first place. If you're struggling to keep up during a "steady" run, then make a deal with yourself to walk for 30 seconds before you try to resume running. Run/walk your way through the workout.

- **Motivation Tip #3: Treat yourself.** As you plan your schedule, also prepare small motivational rewards to which you can treat yourself on your three-level difficulty days. If you complete your workout, then the reward awaits you at home. Consider also rewarding yourself with something really big if you achieve your goal of successfully running your first 5K.

- **Motivation Tip #4: Set yourself up for success.** You must prepare for your workouts. An underprepared workout increases the chances that you'll want to quit your run, because of something you didn't account for that leads you down the path of excuse-making. Here are five questions to ask yourself the night before your workout.

1. How long and how hard will I be running?
2. What route will I choose?
3 What will the temperatures and winds be at the time I plan to run?

4. What time of day will I be running?
5. When will I plan to eat and drink before, during, and after the run?

Knowing the answers to your questions ahead of time should help mitigate the risks of suffering from a possible motivational problem. For example, if you know that the temperature on tomorrow's run will be in the 90s and that you are supposed to do a 30-minute "steady" run, then you decide that you'll run early in the morning. You will bring a water bottle with you, and you'll not take that route with the huge hill. You'll ensure you are well hydrated the night before and that you'll get a good night's sleep and have a light snack in your belly before you head out. **Set yourself up for success by planning properly; don't give your body and mind any excuses to quit when you shouldn't be quitting.**

- **Motivation Tip #5: Find strength in numbers.** Join a local running club and head out with like-minded friends on your workouts. Just having someone there with whom to share your feelings will be a huge help. He/she may offer you advice that you hadn't considered. The same goes for doing harder workouts. Seek out a training buddy with whom you can do your track repeats. Even if he or she is faster than you, just having the company on the track together is the best way to train.

- **Motivation Tip #6: Get pumped!** Have you ever watched a boxer warm up before a match? All the dancing and jumping and head-rolling helps them get pumped up for the main event. You can do the same. Put on some motivational songs before you head out on your run. Jump up and down. Roll your head and throw a couple jabs in the air. Tell yourself some positive affirmations. Be proud of what you are about to set out and do. So many make excuses, but not you. You got this! Another way to get pumped is to watch or read something that motivates you. I've always been drawn to famous runners such as Steve Prefontaine or the great Czech distance runner from the 1950s Emil Zátopek. I've committed quotes of theirs to memory and used to read their biographies before I was gearing up for a big training day.

- **Motivation Tip #7: Establish a routine.** If you're working out, you are successfully shifting your equilibrium. Along those lines, establish new norms. Put your running shoes in a similar place near the door. Organize a set of regular running clothes. Do the same types of prerun warmup routines. Listen to the same music playlist. If you can make running as routine as brushing your teeth or putting on your PJs, then it will be an expected activity that you simply just do, because it's now part of your life.

- **Motivation Tip #8: Run different places.** Though it's essential to establish a routine, it's always a good idea to try out different routes. New courses mean new sights to see. And you can always run a route in reverse—perhaps even alternating one direction on one day and switching it up the next day.

- **Motivation Tip #9: Tell yourself, "Just one more minute."** Remember that there will always be good times and bad times out on the run. If you hit a bad patch, say, "One more minute." Hit the timer on your watch and run for at least 60 seconds more. Just that short period of time could be the time you need for your motivational storm to pass. You can use this same reasoning with landmarks on your run—as in "just one more block" or "until I make it to that big tree."

- **Motivation Tip #10: Write it out.** If you're struggling, write out your feelings in your training log as if it were a diary entry. "Journaling" your thoughts will help you express your emotions. Make sure you also journal on days that you feel strong so that you can revisit these to gain confidence when you are suffering from a dip in morale. Another way to "write it out" is to post about how you are feeling to friends in your social network. A well-placed Facebook post or tweet to the right group can generate the right amount of support to put you at ease.

- **Motivation Tip #11: Listen to your body and take a zero.** There just may be days when you can't seem to get it together. Your body could be telling you something, so listen to it if none of these other tips are helping you. Take the day off and consider taking the next one off as well. Chalk it up to the price of the equilibrium shift, but don't let it sideline you for good. Your motivation will come back—trust me.

Unique Situations

Some of us face special challenges that can prevent us from taking up and then maintaining our running. What follows are some specific situations that you may face and how you can overcome them so that they don't impede you:

Running as a Single Parent

At one point in my life, I was a single dad, caring for my young daughter, and also a 100-mile-a-week marathoner who held a full-time job. It was hardly a cakewalk, but I was so passionate about being able to care for my daughter while experiencing the joy of running that I was able to make it all work. If you are the single parent of a young child, you can, too.

Try these four tips:

1. **Run during your lunch break.** While your child is in daycare or at school and you are at work, see if you can fit in your 30 minutes while others are sitting at their desks eating. Alternatively, ask your boss if it's OK to "block" an hour in your schedule to work out. Many companies encourage their workers to exercise.
2. **Bring your child with you on your workouts, by investing in a jogging stroller.**
3. **Do what you can and follow Training Maxim #1. ("Doing something is better than doing nothing.")** There are many times when the needs of your child will trump your running needs.
4. **Hire a babysitter a few times a week when you are supposed to be doing important hard-effort workouts.** The beauty of the 30-minute running concept is that it won't cost you that much!

Training with a Jogging Stroller

If your child can hold up its own head up (usually six months to a year), then taking them with you on a walk or a run is a possibility. Your best bet in finding the right one is to head to your local running store. Speak to an expert. If you've never tried running while pushing a jogging stroller, then be aware of the following key differences between running solo and running with a companion:

- **Pushing a jog stroller isn't just a leg and lung workout; it's also a back and shoulder workout.** Though many top-of-the-line strollers make the pushing seem effortless thanks to advanced wheel technology, it's still a total-body workout. As such, for every day that you are running with a jog stroller, skip one cross-training day on your schedule.

- **Hills are really hard.** It's challenging enough pushing yourself up a hill, but pushing two people is too much for beginners. Skip all-hill workout days when you are running with a stroller.

- **Keep your child bundled up and occupied.** You may be working out and burning calories, but your precious cargo is sitting in a seat, exposed to the elements. Make sure you have them super snuggled and warm. Carry an extra blanket or two under the stroller.

- **Plan for two people.** Make a checklist for your jogging stroller runs that includes, at minimum, the following: diapers, baby wipes, water bottle, change of clothes, fully charged cellphone in case of emergencies, mini first aid supplies, and extra toys.

- **Run in a safe place.** Avoid busy, noisy, polluted roads, and, if possible, head to a park or open space with paved trails where you and your baby can bond in peace.

- **Check the air in your stroller's tires before you head out on your run.** Many jog strollers leak slowly over time. Do a quick pressure test of the tire's air with your fingers or a tire gauge.

- **Don't do your speed work on the track.** Tracks are typically busy places and many ban strollers outright. Instead, do your speed work on a flat, empty stretch of road or pavement approximately 400 meters in length. Bear in mind that the pace of your faster laps will be much slower.

- **Talk to your child while you are running/walking.** Let them know that you are there. If the two of you are new to jog-stroller running, then expect a period of time where both of you need to adjust to the change.
- **Be prepared to quit the workout.** There are some days when your child won't want to cooperate. If they are crying when you head out, give yourself five minutes and see if they calm down. If not, turn around and head back. You tried (Training Maxim #1).
- **If your child has a routine nap schedule, see if you can fit your runs in during that time.** Many children sleep in the jog stroller.
- **Safety first.** All jog strollers have a harness seatbelt system and many come with a lanyard that you can attach around your wrist in the event that you lose your grip on the stroller. Treat getting your child into the stroller like you were putting them into a car.

The Travelling Runner

If you have a career that has you on the road for up to five days a week, then a lot of the workouts and routines prescribed in this book may seem impossible to achieve. If that's the case, then try out these on-the-road running tips.

- **Do your homework.** This means you should plan your weekly runs in advance. If you have flexibility as to which hotel you will be staying at for work, then do some research. Call the hotel and speak to the concierge. Ask them what the running is like at their hotel. How far are the routes? Are they hilly? How is the traffic around the hotel?

- **Use a treadmill if necessary.** Though I'm not an advocate of treadmill running, I would prefer that you use one if you are staying at a hotel where it's not ideal or safe to go running. Don't just hop on the treadmill and go. Understand how it works and how you can program it to best accommodate your planned workout.

- **Get your walks in at the airport.** Many business travelers get to the airport, sit, and eat. But airports are excellent places to walk around. Go for a walk while you are there. Keep your legs moving. Pulling your carry-on can also act as a mini cross-training exercise for the arms and shoulders.

- **Try to do your workouts in the morning.** Business travel is exhausting. You're sleeping in a strange room. You are in stressful meetings. You are taking cabs and sitting in long meetings. Your best bet to train, therefore, is in the morning. Your chances of putting on your running shoes after returning to your hotel following a series of nine-hour meetings in a conference room with your boss and heading out in the dark night of a strange city are minimal.

- **Don't fall off the "healthy wagon" while you're travelling.** Eating while travelling usually entails sitting in restaurants or binge snacking in the hotel at night. Stay disciplined while on the road. Try to find a coworker who can serve as your workout partner so that you can mutually help one another to live healthy on the road.

- **Plan for the weather.** Look at the forecast where you are travelling and pack accordingly. Besides the temperatures, pay attention to the wind forecast.

- **Find some locals.** Use the Internet to look up some local running stores and cold-call them. Ask them if they have clubs they recommend. Many stores offer group runs. Also ask them for suggestions on decent and safe places to run in the area where you will be staying.

- **Don't take the elevator; climb those stairs.** Hotels typically have fantastic stairwells. Almost no one uses them, so if you want to add some extra difficulty and privacy to your walking workouts, tack on stair repeats. Or you can do stair repeats as a substitute to your hill workouts. Either walk quickly or run up the stairwells. Try to do three to five flights as one repetition.

Chapter 5

SUSTAIN

At this point in the book you should be ready to put all this hard training and discipline into action. This is it: your race day. But before we get too far into the hows and whens of the actual race, we need to dial things back a bit and start at the beginning—to the day that you signed your contract with yourself.

Why did you pick up this book? What motivated you to want to make a change? I'm sure racing has something to do with it, but I doubt that running your first 5K was the only reason to start running.

You want to improve you!

You seek a healthier life and a better outlook. You know that losing weight, eating better, and becoming healthier will improve your confidence and relationships.

Therefore, you first 5K shouldn't be seen as the end of your running pursuits; it's just the beginning.

Ensure that you approach your first race with this kind of curious attitude. You want your first race to be like that first date with your spouse. You want to use it to fall in love with the sport. You don't want it to be a negative, stress-inducing time where you worry about everything. If you set up your first race to be this kind of experience, then there's a good chance you will quit the sport and donate this book to Goodwill. You should want your first 5K to be fun and care-free. So, even though there is a lot of information about the race in this chapter, please keep in mind that first and foremost this event is all about drawing you into a new way of life.

To get the most of your first race, I want you to think about it in three stages: race preparation, race execution, and race introspection.

Race Preparation

Up to now, you've been preparing for some unknown race on some undefined course. About five or six weeks to go before your targeted race date, you begin selecting the race that will be best suited for you. The good news is that in most parts of the urbanized world, 5Ks are a commonly held weekend event. But the experience you can have in a 5K can vary greatly. If not properly advertised and promoted, some small 5K races may have as few as five to thirty people taking part. Conversely, there are large-city 5Ks, usually held in conjunction with other events like half marathons or marathons that can have participation numbers in the thousands.

As a beginner who seeks to fall in love with the sport, I suggest you find a 5K that's fun. While doing a small-town event with twenty like-minded people may be enjoyable, it probably won't be something that you'll want to do as your first race. Small 5Ks are typically isolated affairs with hardly anyone there to cheer you on and oftentimes don't have road closures or any kind of decent support that will make the event seem special. But before you get into the details of which race is right for you, you need to first know where to look for a good race. Here are some sources to help you narrow your search for that optimal event:

- **Talk to your shoe expert.** If you've made a friend at your local running store who got you into your original pair of trainers, then hit them up for advice. Ask them to point you to a good first-time 5K. Explain what your goals are and your progress thus far.

- **Ask some of your fellow runners for ideas.** If you're taking part in group runs or workouts on a regular basis and have established a rapport with more-seasoned runners, then ask them to list their favorite races.

- **Check the Internet.** The Web can be a tremendous asset for race research. Just Google your city, "5K," and the date you want to run the race, and you should get back a lot of options.

- **Write to the race director.** Almost all races have a "race director." This person, usually an underpaid, overworked runner, is responsible for everything about the race—from registration to advertising to timing. If you find a race on the Web that looks like a good fit, then feel free to contact them via email to learn more. Ask them about the course—is it "fast" (meaning usually if it's flat with few turns), what kind of crowd support there will be, and if she or he considers it a good race for beginners. If you are planning to walk the course, then ask them if there is a minimum cut-off time where runners who don't make it to the end at that time will be asked to stop. I would strongly advise that you not select your first 5K with a minimum cut-off time as it might put unnecessary pressure on you to finish the race at a pace you aren't comfortable with.

- **Volunteer.** A good way to find the perfect race for you is to volunteer at a 5K. Race directors are always looking for help. Typically, volunteers help with traffic control or prerace registration, which is an excellent way to experience a race close up without having to actually run it. Besides getting to know local runners, you can also get a feel for the course, as most local 5Ks are held on the same or similar stretches of road.

Race-Selection Criteria

If you've got a few good race candidates in mind, you'll want to narrow down your search to find the most ideal 5K fit for your needs so that you can have the best possible first experience. Here are some key criteria that can help you in your search:

- **The course.** This is probably the most important element of your first race. If you end up selecting a difficult course with lots of hills or turns, you are going to have a harder time. A good 5K course for a beginner should be flat and fast. The fewer hills, the better. Another thing for which you'll want to be on the lookout is the course layout. Is there one loop? Does it comprise several loops? Is it an "out and back"? An "out and back" course means that you typically run about 1.5 miles out to a cone or line and then turn around and head back. I would discourage you from these courses, because it's challenging mentally and physically to turn around and run back to the start. For your first 5K, try doing a single-loop course. This means that all landmarks are new and you aren't seeing the same thing again. The more "fresh" the views, the more energy you can get when you are struggling. Stay clear, also, of two- or three-loop "criterium" courses, as the temptation will be high to drop out after the first lap.

- **The support.** Races run with no crowd support can be lonely affairs. When you are running your first 5K, you are going to want lots of people on the sidelines cheering you on. You are going to want music, cheerleaders, performers, and finish-line announcers who call out to people when they are coming across the line. You'll want to high-five strangers and hear their words of support. Consider finding a popular, loud, rambunctious first 5K. Don't run your first race in a vacuum. You will be feeding off the energy, so the more that exists, the better. Another aspect of race-day support is how well prepared the race organizers are to handle the crowds. You can contact the race director beforehand and ask them support questions, such as: How many water stops does the race offer? Have they ever run out of water before? Are energy gels or drinks offered at their water stops? Are there any portable toilets available to runners mid-course? Finally, do some investigation into crowd management and control. Where are runners supposed to park before the race?
- **A charity you can get behind.** Most 5Ks are fundraisers for charities. If you have a specific cause to which you already donate, then see if they host a 5K in which you can partake. If you are already passionate about the cause going into it, then it

will motivate you even more to finish when you are out on the roads. Some races also offer you the ability to run as part of a charity team. This is a great way to raise money for your favorite cause while motivating you to stay focused on your training.

- **The finisher medal.** The first 5K that you finish should be something that you cherish for a lifetime—a true and memorable achievement that is worthy of the spotlight. As such, understand if the race gives out a finisher medal. If they don't, then perhaps try to find one that hands out such an award, because you are most likely going to hang this medal on your wall as a mark of pride and achievement.

- **The weather.** The majority of 5Ks allow you to sign up on race day. You can usually preregister in advance, but even though you can save money doing this, I would strongly encourage you not to do that. Your first 5K shouldn't be something that takes part in gale-force winds or a driving snowstorm or in sweltering heat and humidity. Wait until a few days before the race, when weather forecasts are more accurate, to make your decision. Also, think about running your first 5K in a location that has conditions similar to where you've been training so that your body doesn't have to acclimate. If you live and train in Florida, for example, don't decide to fly to Anchorage, Alaska and do your first race as part of a longer family vacation to the great northern state.

What to Expect on Race Day and How to Plan for Success

Once you've selected your race, it's time to plan for success on the big day. If you've never run a road race before, it's helpful to know how races typically operate. Some large races require online prerace registration, while others allow you to sign up before the start on the day of the race (sometimes for a higher fee). Once you are registered for a race, you will need to pick up your "bib," which is your race number that you pin to your t-shirt. Most races these days also provide you with a chip that you thread through your shoelace or attach with zip ties. This chip registers with sensor mats that the race director places at the start and finish as well as any checkpoints along the way. Chip timing is a great way to allow you to know how fast you ran the race, taking into account the time you actually crossed the start and finish line, and not including how long it took you to make it to the starting line. For crowded races, this could take minutes, so wearing a chip should give you peace of mind that you don't need to fight your way towards to front in order to log an accurate race time.

Besides the chip mats, the finish-line funnel is another item of which you should be aware. Some races set these up right at the end as a way to channel runners at the finish so that race staff can log results in an organized fashion and provide finishers with their medals. Finally, be on the lookout for the fluid stations. These are typically tables set up at points along the course with cups of water for runners to take. The cups can sometimes also contain Gatorade, and some races offer energy snacks (bars or gels).

At the finish, most races turn into parties with music, food, and drinks. Top finishers receive awards, and you can get your gear if you checked it in before the start.

With a good understanding of what to expect, it's time to do some proper race-day planning. This requires five key steps:

Step 1: Know the course. There will be a lot of surprises that you encounter on the day of your first race. Many will be unpreventable, but not knowing the course should not be one of them. You can get to know the course in advance of your race by going to the race's website. If the site doesn't have the course listed, write to the race director to find out. Once you know the course, the best thing you can do is train on it—especially on the last mile. On race day, this will be the part of the course where you will be working the hardest. Your legs will be hurting and your lungs may be starved for oxygen. If you can memorize this section, then there won't be any surprises, like a small uphill portion or a sudden change in direction that could throw you off when you are exhausted. Another way to know the course is to get an elevation profile of it. Many larger 5Ks offer this on their website. The elevation profile will show you the ups and downs you will face on race day. Ask yourself: How many hills are there? Where in the race will I be encountering them? How large are the hills? Knowing about the hills will allow you to plot how to allocate your energy in the race itself. Print out the course map and add it to your training journal. Write out the hills on your course map and circle anything else such as where the water stops will be and where to expect cheer zones or quieter stretches. Use this course map as your guide to the race itself. Another important aspect of the course is knowing where you will park and how you will get home. If you can take public transportation to the race, that would be ideal, as the stress (and cost) of finding public parking can cause unnecessary worry and distract you from focusing on your race.

Step 2: Know the weather. What are the expected highs and lows for the day? What will the temperatures be an hour before you are running the race, when you are running the race, and an hour after? How about the dew point? Will it be humid? Check the wind speed and direction and know where you will be facing a headwind on the course so you can mentally prepare to have to work harder there.

Step 3: Make a checklist. The last thing you need to worry about on race day is forgetting something important like your ID or extra clothes. I like to tell my athletes to use the back of their course map as a race-day checklist where they write out the things they need to remember to bring and do. Here is a good starting point for your checklist:

- Identification
- Change of clothes. Put these in a sealed, dry bag in the event of rain during the race.
- Course map in a ziplock bag
- Small hand sanitizer bottle
- Extra safety pins
- Vaseline and Band-Aids
- Refillable water bottle
- Light snack: bagel, granola bar, or energy bars
- Extra socks sealed in a ziplock bag
- Running hat and, if it's cold out, a spare knit cap
- For winter races, some chemical hand warmers
- Small amount of cash for emergencies
- Warmup clothes

Step 4: Take your prerace rest, meals, and sleep seriously. You've worked very hard for this day, so make sure that you are ready. Being ready means preparing your body to be in the best shape possible to meet your goal on the day of the race. Race day is a "hard" training day, so that means you must rest. The day before the race, put your feet up and relax. You will probably be nervous, so try to do something that lets your mind wander. Go see a movie or spend time with your family. The day before, have a large carbohydrate-heavy lunch like spaghetti or lasagna. Pay attention to your hydration throughout the day. Monitor your urine color. Carry your refillable water bottle with you and ensure you are drinking often. Have a light dinner and try to get to bed early. Lay out all your equipment before you turn in so that you aren't scrambling in the morning, looking for misplaced things.

Step 5: Practice positive thinking and visualization. The day before your race, you need to stay 100 percent positive. Take some time to look through all your notes in your log. Read about your ups and your downs. Focus especially on the times in your training where you may have doubted yourself but prevailed. Tomorrow's event will be challenging. Know that there may be moments during the event where you will want to step off the course and give up, but you must press on. Watch or read something inspirational like the movie *Chariots of Fire*. If you've been meditating as part of your training, dedicate an entire session the day before to visualizing about your race day. Tell yourself the following things:

- I'm proud of what I've been able to accomplish.
- I am thankful that I am healthy enough to take part in this event. I've faced my doubts and fears and overcome them.
- I know I will experience pain and suffering while I'm racing, but this is part of my equilibrium shift. When I am experiencing pain and suffering during the race, I will tell myself that it's part of my positive evolution as a stronger person.
- The finish line will arrive sooner than I think.

As part of your visualization, imagine yourself as a strong person during the race. Imagine that each mile will feel better than the last. Think about the finisher's medal around your neck. Hear the spectators on either side of you. Try to visualize the course. On any uphill section, imagine you powering up them with the same strength that you've used on your hill repeats. On any downhill part, think about catching your breath and recovering your energy. After you've reached the halfway point, tell yourself that from there, it will only feel easier, because you are almost done. Now, imagine the finish line in the distance. You see it getting closer. The crowd gets louder. Only a few more feet now. You cross the line and pump your fist. You've made it. You will make it tomorrow. You will prevail, because you deserve to prevail.

Race Execution

In order to make sure that your race is an enjoyable experience, you have to first realize that it isn't a "final exam." Final exams are stressful affairs. Everything seems to be riding on the results. This does not apply to your race! First, know that races come and go. There will always be another race around the corner for you. Though you will be doing everything you can to meet your goal, there may be circumstances that come into play that you can't control. **Don't pin everything onto how you performed in this one event.** What you want from your race is to fall in love with the sport, so having fun is what matters most. Showing up on race day—that's the one thing that you must do. To run your best possible race, there are some things you can do to optimize your performance:

- **Make sure you're warmed up.** Get to the race at least 45 minutes before the start and walk or jog for 10 minutes right before the race's start. Warmed-up legs are the best way to prevent injury to them.

- **Use the bathroom.** The last thing you need to worry about on race day is having to use the loo. As soon as you get to the race location, scout out the toilets.

- **At the start, look down at your feet to make sure your laces are double-knotted.** The last think you need to worry about is an untied shoelace while you are in the middle of a large crowd of excited people.

- **Control your early pace.** Race starting lines are exciting places full of energy and excitement. Try to contain this. Once the starting gun goes off, do not sprint. Your first few minutes should not feel like the "hard" lap that you ran as part of your speed work. If this is your first 5K, then rule out going fast altogether. There is nothing wrong with walking at the start (or during the entire race). Don't feel "peer pressure" to run fast. Conserve your energy. Keep telling yourself, "Go slow." And get used to all these people zooming past you. Your instinct will be to take off with them, but resist that temptation.

- **Feed off the crowd.** Use the spectators to help you along the way. If this is your first 5K, tell people that by writing it on your race shirt so that you can get some extra high fives. Any time you spend running up to people and searching out these accolades is worth it.

- **Find a buddy.** After the first mile, you will most likely be running with people who are at the same fitness level with you. Strike up a short conversation with someone around you. Tell them of your goal. Ask them what they hope to achieve. There is strength in numbers out there on the race course. Having a buddy to push you along and console you when you aren't feeling good can be a tremendous help. Conversely, if your buddy is struggling, use some of your energy to encourage them. Give them a pep talk. This positive energy can help you with your own pace and even serve to distract you from any of your own aches and pains.

- **Practice smart refueling.** Fluid stations can be chaotic places. Some runners try to grab water while running by and this can lead to lots of spills, slips, and confusion. If you are going to grab a cup of water, do it while walking. Make eye contact with the volunteer and don't drink the water in front of the station. Instead, keep walking and gradually sip the water as you walk. Gradual fluid replenishment is a good way to prevent sudden abdominal cramping. It's also safer since you will be drinking your water out of the "line of fire" of thirsty runners around you. Another thing you can do at a fluid stop on a hot day is to grab two cups of water. Use one cup of water to drink and with the other one, pour it over your head to cool you down. If you are wearing a racing hat, then pour the water into your hat and put the hat back on.

- **Use your fellow racers to shield you from the wind.** There is nothing wrong with letting other runners on the course block the wind for you. If your race is on a blustery day, then look for a "pack" of racers that is going your pace and get in behind them when you're encountering a stretch of the course with a strong headwind. Feel free to return the wind-shielding favor for any stretch of the race where you feel strong.

- **Do what you did in training: walk when it hurts.** When you struggled with your runs in training, you hopefully resorted to walking breaks. Do the same thing at the race. If you feel like you can't keep running, set your watch to countdown for 30 seconds and tell yourself that you will at least run for that time. Sometimes, all you need is a little goal like this to get a second wind. If after 30 seconds you feel like you can't go on, then take a walk break. Walk for two minutes and run for two minutes. If you can't alternate between two minutes of walking/running, then do two minutes of walking and one minute of running. These walk/run breaks can help give you little periods of rest and recovery between the harder segments. You'll also notice that these kinds of pace changes can help shake you out of a mental slump and make the race move along faster.

- **Power through the hills.** One of the reasons I have you training on hills in your workouts is to learn how to summit them come race day. If you encounter a long or steep hill on the race course, remember to pump your arms to get some momentum going. Use the same mental techniques you used on the hills in your training. Tell yourself that the hill will come to pass. One step at a time. You can do it. Think about the "payoff" in the form of a welcoming downhill section later in the course when you will be able to cruise and recover. Hills are always tough, but they don't last forever. Your training has made you "hill-resistant."

- **Sprint to the finish line.** Once you see the finish line in sight, go for it. If you don't have anything left in your legs, then don't worry about it. But if you do, that short adrenaline burst will carry you into the home stretch. Just suddenly changing the pace like this can also be a good way to shake things up. Just seeing the finish line can be an exhilarating experience. Give the spectators something to cheer about.

- **Remember the #1 rule in racing.** I tell my athletes that there is only one rule with races and that is that there will be good miles and bad miles, but the good miles can and do come after bad miles. Most runners out on the race course think that once they start feeling bad, they will only start to feel worse. They convince themselves that the only thing they can do once their legs hurt and their lungs burn is to do damage control. If you are starting to feel bad, do a quick "system check." Ask yourself the following questions:

- How are my feet feeling? Can I feel my toes? Are my arches sore? Are my feet rubbing my shoes anywhere?
- How are my legs feeling? Any aches or pains in the calves, thighs, knees, or quads?
- How are my lungs? Am I breathing heavy? Is my breathing pained?
- How is my mouth feeling? Is it dry? Am I thirsty?
- How are my arms, back, and shoulders feeling? Am I clenching my fists?
- How is my stride? Am I feeling bent over or am I feeling straight?
- How is my head feeling? Is my mind still in the race? Do I feel confident that I will make my goal?

After your "system check" try to understand the pain points. Why are you having them? Then realize that you can do something about this. All is not lost. Start by telling yourself that you are going to turn around these bad thoughts and feelings, and make the negative a positive. Then immediately start righting any wrongs that you identify in your system check. Here are some examples of how to alleviate your mid-race aches and pains:

- If your feet are bothering you, then take a moment to step to the side of the course and adjust your shoes. Perhaps the tongue of the shoe has slipped or your laces are either too loose or too tight.

- If your legs are bothering you, touch your pain points and give them a light massage. Use positive thoughts to imagine your touch helping ward off the pain and doubt.

- If your breathing is pained, then you are most likely running too fast. Slow down. If you are trying to run/walk or run, then just transition to a walk until you can get your breathing back under control.

- If you're thirsty, take a drink from your water bottle or plan to drink at the next water stop.

- Arm, neck, and shoulder pain typically means you are clenching your fists. Consciously relax your hands. Make sure no fingers are touching.

- Fix your stride. The more we fatigue, the more likely we are to "sit in the bucket" while running—which means hunching our backs and bending our heads down. Focus on your form by imagining that a racer ahead of you has lassoed a rope around your hips and is pulling them forward.

- If you are getting doubts about the race, immediately think positive thoughts. Think about how far you've run. Think about all those workouts you've done to prepare for this big day. If you've found a running buddy out on the race course, share your doubts with him or her.

- If you have to use the bathroom, find a portable toilet. The time it takes to deal with nature is worth the sacrifice more than dealing with the discomfort, worry, or potential embarrassment of trying to "hold it."

Postrace Introspection

If you successfully complete your first 5K or clock a personal-best time, then the only thing with which you should be concerning yourself is celebration. Wear that medal with pride! Make sure, though, that you don't forget to do a good 5- to 10-minute cooldown and some light stretching. If you aren't successful in your first attempt at a 5K, then don't despair. As I've written earlier: races aren't final exams. There will always be another race around the corner for you. Regardless how the race went, take time when you get home to do some introspection about how you felt. Use your log to write out the following data points:

- Race name:
- Race date:
- Race location:
- Race-day temperature and winds:
- Time and place:

Then write out what went well about the race. What did you like? Did you achieve any milestones? Additionally, jot down what you didn't like. These are key lessons learned that you'd like to avoid next time. Try to focus on things that you can control when you next race. For example, perhaps you didn't pack warmly enough. Or, you drank too much water in the first mile and cramped up in the second mile.

If You Didn't Achieve Your Race-Day Goal

Do Not Beat Yourself Up

Negative thoughts about why you didn't achieve what you wanted are never helpful. Be constructive with your introspection. Write down three things with which you struggled during the race and how you can address these in training. Think about how each area of your "system check" felt. Did any one area of your body feel worse than another? Perhaps you ran a course with a steep hill and your legs were extremely tired after reaching the top of it, so you could conclude that you need to do more hill training next time. Here are some typical factors that prevent people from achieving their race-day goals:

- **You didn't do the work in training.** Look at your training log. Did you do the workouts you were supposed to do? Did you take any excessively long "rest" days?

- **You didn't do the right kind of work in training.** Did you complete the hard workouts you were supposed to do? Did you run the hills and do the longer runs and walks?

- **You did too much work.** Look at the workouts you did in the few days leading up to the race. Perhaps you were overtrained and tired going into the race?

- **You didn't fuel properly.** It could be that you didn't eat enough the day before. Or perhaps you ate too soon before the race, causing you to cramp to the point that your sides hurt too much to continue. Look at fueling as a suspect if you struggled with low energy or if you felt any abdominal pain.

- **You didn't conserve your energy.** Perhaps you got too excited at the start and went out too aggressively in the first mile? Think about how your breathing felt during the race. If you were out of breath in the early stages, you probably were running too fast. The best way to learn from this lesson is to race again. As you gain more race-day experience, you will understand how to control your pace and allocate your energy. You can also practice this in your speed work training sessions. Chapter 6 explains some more advanced, race-pace training options that you can incorporate in your training when you prepare for your next race.

- **The negative side of your mind got the better of you.** You may have just had a bad day and decided to step off the course and "live to fight another day." We can't always be performing at 100 percent. Watch an elites race and you will see plenty of DNFs (did not finish) going on. Discretion is the better form of valor, so just because you quit the race doesn't detract in any bit from your character or your being as a runner. Just don't make that one bad race day transform you into writing off the sport altogether. Remember, it's not about the race; it's about your positive mental and physical transformation.

- **You had a race-day malfunction.** The early parts of this chapter should prepare you to prevent most of the bad things that can come your way, but there are so many variables that could go wrong. Perhaps you twisted your ankle five minutes before the start or you ate something that didn't agree with you in the morning. Whatever these malfunctions are, just be aware that they can happen to anyone. Olympic gold medalists experience them, and so can you. If you experience a race-day malfunction, just grin and bear it. Think about how you can minimize the risk the next time you race and remember that races come and go and that another 5K is just around the corner for you.

If You Did Achieve Your Race-Day Goal

Congratulations!

Take your signed contract and frame it on your wall. Go out and celebrate. But still spend some time on introspection and try to give yourself an honest critique. Organize your thoughts about the race into things you'd like to keep doing and things you should improve on. Take a few days of rest and then think about your next goals as a 5K runner. If this was your first time completing a 5K while walking it, then make it a goal to do your next 5K on a run/walk. Take a look at the other more advanced schedules in Chapter 6 and try those out as you begin a new training cycle to achieve your next goal.

Chapter 6

THRIVE

At some point in your running career, you may want to take it to the next level. This chapter is all about how to progress in the sport, running further and faster than you've ever run before. The schedules in this chapter cover doubling the race distance—from 5K to 10K.

Before you get too far into this chapter, though, I'd like you to think about why you want to move up in distance. Just because you've run a few 5Ks may not mean that you should try to go longer. Many professional runners spend years perfecting their craft in the shorter distances, and there is nothing wrong with never racing a distance longer than 5K. At a minimum, I think you should do at least three 5Ks, with one done running the entire distance (no walking) before you contemplate "moving up" in race distance.

The 10K is an entirely different event. At double the 5K distance, there is a lot more that you have to endure on the roads, tracks, and trails. Your legs have to be stronger. "Stronger" means that your legs have more muscle fibers and can run longer thanks to wider capillaries and a "stronger" heart that can deliver oxygenated blood to these capillaries efficiently.

Therefore, training for your first 10K isn't going to be the same as the 5K. This new distance means doing five things differently:

Difference #1: Workouts Longer Than 30 Minutes

This book is primarily about working out for 30 minutes or less, but if you are going to double the distance, then you will need to double some of your workout times. As you will see in the example 10K training schedule, I have tried to keep the majority of your workouts at 30 minutes or less, but there may be an occasion when you need to exceed this time period. If you are just starting to experiment with running longer than 30 minutes, then you need to be mindful of not trying to "bite off more than you can chew." In other words, ease into your longer workouts. A good rule of thumb is to increase your workout times by no more than 10 to 20 percent per week. So if your longest workout has been 30 minutes, then make sure you don't increase that by more than three to five minutes in the subsequent training week. The body doesn't like sudden changes, so it can be risky to try to overachieve with these longer workouts. The last think you want is to get injured in your second week because you tried to run for an hour, so err on the side of caution with your workout.

Difference #2: Goal-Pace Workouts

By the time you are ready to move into 10Ks, you should be running your 5Ks, so achieving personal bests is probably important to you. Additionally, the longer the race, the higher the chances are that you can make a mistake with your pacing—usually going out too fast too early. This is where goal-pace workouts come in. They will teach you how to "internalize and memorize" paces that you hope to run on race day. This means you will be training your mind and body, gradually, to get used to speed at the edges of your comfort zone.

Difference #3: The Introduction of the Long Run

Long runs are excellent ways to build leg strength. Though most runners consider "long runs" as longer than 90 minutes, the 60-minute runs I've prescribed in this sample schedule should count—especially if you've never run or walked for that much time.

Difference #4: Fueling

The longer you are out on the race course, the more important your water and carbohydrate consumption become. You will need to be drinking more water before, during, and after your 10K workouts. You will also need to increase your caloric consumption with every extra minute of workout time you complete during your training week.

Difference #5: Speed Bursts

Think of the speed burst workouts as short injections of speed to break up the monotony of a run and give your body an extra challenge. Suddenly "switching gears" can make your runs go by quicker and are also fun. By training to do bursts, you will become mentally stronger, gaining confidence that you can run faster if need be. Speed bursts help train you for that "finishing kick" and work different sets of fast-twitch muscles than you are used to working when you run slower. This is a new training concept for you and if not done with some caution and gradualism, could result in injury, because of the sudden demands on the legs and feet to work at a pace they aren't prepared for. To account for this risk, you will see that the schedule has you doing these workouts with some added precautions like easing into the speed bursts and doing bursts for very short periods of time.

All these differences aside, one thing will remain constant as you try to attain your next running milestone: the great equilibrium shift. After you've got a few 5Ks under your belt, they will seem easier. You will probably begin to feel comfortable running so far. You will feel confident with your new routine. But when you decide to double the distance, you have to expect to encounter those same pesky resistant forces. You will encounter all the same challenges that you faced when you initially donned your first pair of trainers. You will want to quit. You'll doubt yourself. You'll be tired and question why you are doing what you are doing. You'll get angry, frustrated, and irritated.

Quitting is the easy response to the equilibrium shift, but you have to remember that change is never easy. Shifting your equilibrium comes with a price, but that price is well worth it. Keep going. Those long runs and strange goal-pace workouts will be hard at first, but your body will adapt.

A Sample 10K Training Plan

Starting on page 135, you'll find an example plan that you can follow to complete your first 10K. This plan is for first-timers who want to finish the race on a run or a run/walk. Unlike the 5K plans, there is just one plan here. It's more of a sample than a prescriptive guide, and I'd suggest that you read through it to understand the key principles and tailor it to your own needs. The same basic workout types that you completed in the 5K plan are still applicable here, but with the following three additions:

- **Long Run: Medium-Intensity Workout.** This is simply a workout longer than 30 minutes. The pace for this workout should be as slow as you need it to be. Walking is OK, so too is run/walking. For this workout, bring water with you and also a light snack. Make sure you've done good course and weather research in advance of your first "long run" so that you don't accidentally select a route with steep hills that will make "going the distance" even more of a challenge. Or you end up accidentally doing your "long run" during the hottest or windiest period of the day. These workouts are considered to be "hard" because you will be going farther than you've ever run in your life, so take these workouts seriously. Make sure you're adequately rested and have paid extra attention to your hydration before, during, and after the run.

- **Goal Pace: Hard-Intensity Workout.** This is the only workout described here that deviates from this book's time-based construct. It is given in terms of how many miles you should run at your goal pace. For all these workouts, do at least a 5-minute warmup and cooldown. To determine your unique "goal pace" for your miles, you should think about what time you hope to run. If this is your first 10K, then double your 5K personal best time and add at least five minutes to that finishing time. Then determine the minutes-per-mile average of that time to determine your unique "goal pace." Here's an example: if your fastest 5K is 32 minutes, then you should aim to run your first 10K in 70 minutes (32 minutes × 2 = 64 + six extra minutes). Using a pace calculator from the Web, you can see that your race pace for a 10K in 70 minutes would be 11 minutes and 15 seconds per mile. You can do your goal-pace workouts on a track, knowing that roughly four laps equals a mile (a metric track is 400 meters and there are 1,609.34 meters in a mile).

To continue this example, if your goal pace workout is to be two miles, then you should run eight laps in a little less than 22 minutes and 30 seconds. Precise times aren't important for these workouts. What is important is that you are running at a pace that you feel seems sustainable for the entire 6.2 miles that comprises the 10K event.

- **Speed Bursts: Medium-Intensity Workout.** These workouts require you to suddenly increase the pace of your run. The sample schedule has them listed in terms of how many bursts you should do, the amount of time that you should be doing the burst, and how much time between bursts you should take for "steady" running. If you've never done a speed burst before then make sure that you are sufficiently warmed up and that you "ease" into them. A good rule of thumb for how fast you should run your "burst" is how fast you ran your speed work laps in your 5K training, but do not get hung up about having to run a predetermined pace for each one. What's important is the pace change stimulus you are providing to your mind and body. If you feel the need to walk after your speed burst, that is OK, but try to pick up a slow jog after a minute or two of rest. Another good idea for doing speed burst training is to run these workouts with a training partner—especially someone who has done one before can help you understand how to do these so that you are able to complete all the bursts.

Sample 12-Week Beginner 10K Schedule

Do this schedule if you have already completed a 5K race and feel comfortable training to race a longer distance.

Week 1's Purpose: Base Building

Mon	Tues	Wed	Thurs	Fri	Sat	Sun
Easy, Walk, 30	Rest	Easy, Walk, 30	Rest	Easy, Walk, 40	Rest	Easy, Walk, 40

Week 2's Purpose: Base Building

Mon	Tues	Wed	Thurs	Fri	Sat	Sun
Rest	Medium, Walk/Run, 20 (3/2)	Rest	Medium, Steady Running, 30	Rest	Medium, Steady Running, 30	Rest

Week 3's Purpose: Rest and Recover

Mon	Tues	Wed	Thurs	Fri	Sat	Sun
Cross-Train • Plank 3 × 30 secs • Standing Bicycle Crunches 3 × 10 • 10 Burpees	Medium, Walk/Run, 30 (3/2)	Easy, Walk, 40	Rest	Medium, Steady Running, 30	Rest	Cross-Train • Plank 3 × 30 secs • Standing Bicycle Crunches 3 × 10 • 10 Burpees

Week 4's Purpose: Base Building

Mon	Tues	Wed	Thurs	Fri	Sat	Sun
Rest	Medium, Long Run, 40	Rest	Medium, Walk/Run, 30 (2/3)	Rest	Rest	Medium, Long Run, 40

Week 5's Purpose: Base Building

Mon	Tues	Wed	Thurs	Fri	Sat	Sun
Rest	Medium, Speed Bursts, 30 (3 bursts of 30 secs each with 2 minutes between bursts)	Rest	Medium, Speed Bursts, 30 (3 bursts of 1 minute each with 2 minutes between bursts)	Rest	Medium, Long Run, 40	Rest

Week 6's Purpose: Hills or Speed Work

Mon	Tues	Wed	Thurs	Fri	Sat	Sun
Medium, Walk/ Run, 30 (2/3)	Rest	Hard, Hills • 15 minutes, Walk • 4 Hills • 5-minute Cooldown	Rest	Hard, Hills • 15 minutes, Walk • 5 Hills • 5-minute Cooldown	Rest	Medium, Walk/Run, 30 (2/3)

Week 7's Purpose: Rest and Recover

Mon	Tues	Wed	Thurs	Fri	Sat	Sun
Rest	Medium, Steady Running, 20	Rest	Cross-Train • Plank 3 × 30 secs • Standing Bicycle Crunches 4 × 10 • 15 burpees	Rest	Medium, Steady Running, 20	Rest

Week 8's Purpose: Base Building

Mon	Tues	Wed	Thurs	Fri	Sat	Sun
Rest	Hard, Goal Pace • 10 minutes- Warmup • ½ mile Goal Pace • 10 minutes Cooldown	Rest	Medium, Steady Running, 30	Rest	Medium, Long Run, 50	Rest

Week 9's Purpose: Base Building

Mon	Tues	Wed	Thurs	Fri	Sat	Sun
Medium, Steady Running, 30	Rest	Medium, Steady Running, 30	Cross-Train • Standing Bicycle Crunches 3 × 20 • 8 Burpees	Rest	Medium, Long Run, 45	Rest

Week 10's Purpose: Hills or Speed Work

Mon	Tues	Wed	Thurs	Fri	Sat	Sun
Hard, Speed Work • 5 minute, Warmup • 1 Steady lap • 4 Hard laps with 3 minute Rest between • 5 minute Cooldown	Rest	Medium, Steady Running, 30	Rest	Hard, Goal Pace • 10 minutes, Warmup • 1 mile Goal Pace • 10 minutes Cooldown	Rest	Medium, Steady Running, 30

Week 11's Purpose: Base Building

Mon	Tues	Wed	Thurs	Fri	Sat	Sun
Rest	Medium, Long Run, 50	Rest	Medium, Steady, 30	Rest	Medium, Speed Bursts, 30 (3 bursts of 30 secs each with 2 minutes between bursts)	Medium, Steady Running, 30

Week 12's Purpose: Rest and Recover

Mon	Tues	Wed	Thurs	Fri	Sat	Sun
Cross-Train • Standing Bicycle Crunches 3 × 20 • Plank 3 × 45 secs • 10 Burpees	Rest	Medium, Steady Running, 20	Rest	Medium, Steady Running, 15	Rest	Race Day!

Dos and Don'ts on Race Day

Doing your first race that is twice the distance may seem intimidating, but remember that if you've put in the training, you will have most likely covered a good part of this distance during your 1-hour run. Reread the race section in the previous chapter, and take into account some extra dos and don'ts for your first 6.2-mile run.

Do: Make sure you complete your long runs in training. If you aren't able to run at least 50 to 60 minutes, then there's a good chance that you won't be comfortable covering the 10K distance on race day. Do not skimp on your "long runs." Do them, even if it means walking for parts of the workout.

Don't: Go out too fast on race day. If you get caught up in the race excitement and run at your 5K pace in the first mile, then there's a good chance that you will go into oxygen debt early and never be able to recover. Tell yourself to go slow and let people race past you early on.

Do: Buckle up for a bumpy ride. Even though you've trained for the race, doubling your distance at a faster pace will certainly come with some challenging moments—both mental and physical. Be ready for the "bad" miles and don't forget the #1 rule in racing: *there will be good miles and bad miles, but good miles can and do come after bad miles.* If you hit a bad patch, slow it down and even do some walk/run periods to recover.

Do: Take your time at fueling stops. 10K races typically have more water and fueling stations than what you are used to. You should be hydrating more and to avoid any cramps out on the course, ensure you're taking your time to drink or eat. Don't drink while on the run. Take a water cup and walk with it past the water station, drinking small gulps. Then give yourself at least a 1- or 2-minute walk break after you've refueled before you resume your run.

Don't: Race for time. Your first 10K should be about nothing more than completing the distance. Don't stress about running at a prescribed pace—even the "goal pace" you used in training. If you want to challenge yourself, then try to complete the 6.2-mile distance with as few walk breaks as possible.

Do: Think about buying a pair of shoes for racing. Elite runners do their 5K and 10K races in "flats," which are extremely light shoes with minimal support and cushioning. *You don't need these. In fact, I would strongly discourage you from buying a pair of racing flats, because your legs and feet most likely aren't conditioned to cover the distance and time with such little arch support and cushioning.* However, you may want to think about buying an extra pair of racing shoes. These shoes should be the exact same brand and size that you train in. The reason for these "racing shoes" is purely mental. Having a "use only on race day" pair in your closet will make your first 10K that much more special. Putting on these new shoes will empower you. Also, since they have little to no wear and tear, they should feel fresh and welcoming.

Don't: Try new things during the race. Your first foray into 10 kilometers should not be a grand experiment. A long time ago, I ran the Miami Marathon in the hopes of achieving a PR. After walking through the prerace expo, I decided to buy a pair of "minimalist" marathon racing flats. On the day of the race, I didn't wear my usual pair of flats in which I had been training and opted instead to wear this new pair of fancy shoes. I ended up running a horrible time and had to limp my way to the finish line with blistered and bruised feet. The moral of this story is that you should not try experimenting with anything on the day of your first

10K race. Don't try new energy bars or gels and certainly don't buy shoes the day before the race. Your race should be nothing more than an extension of the consistency that you established in all your training. Go with what worked to get you to the starting line and save dabbling and experimentation for a different day.

Do: Commit to trying another race. Even if your first 10K is less than ideal, know that, like anything, it will improve with practice. Doubling the distance is no easy feat and it may take a few tries to get it right. Like the 5K, do a long amount of post-race introspection and try to locate trends in your performance that can be improved with more training. For example, if your first 10K wasn't a success because of a course with several late-race hills, then focus your next block of training on hills. Fit several extra weeks of hills into your schedule and make sure that you feel confident that you've improved that training gap before you attempt your second 10K. Alternately, you could instead choose a less challenging course in your next 10K attempt.

Turning into a Competitor

At some point in your running journey, you may experience the thrill of competition. After you've got a few races under your belt and you've started making gains, improving your personal best times, you may want to experience more from your races—actually seeking to run faster than those around you. What follows are several tips to consider if you want to dabble in some friendly competition:

- **Find the right people to race.** At the start of the race, strike up conversations with those around you. As a beginner, you should be further back from the starting line than the faster racers. Look around you and see if you can locate runners who appear to be in the same shape that you are in. Some larger races have "corrals" where runners are grouped by ability. Races also have informal or formal "pace groups" with a more experienced leader who has committed to run a prescribed goal pace for the race. Find these runners of similar ability and ask them what their goals are. If they are out to run a similar time, then stick near them and see if you can keep them in your sights during the race. Having a group of people to race will improve your chances of running a personal best.

- **Use a few mental strategies out on the course.** If you find yourself in a foot race with some competitors out on the course, there are a few things you can do to gain a mental edge over them. If you watch Olympic runners compete on the roads, you usually see a large pack of runners. Typically the "front runner" is not the person who eventually wins the race. These front runners are usually setting the pace for the race. Let them do the hard work of wind shielding and dictating the pace. You can slip in behind your rival and let them lead while you stay a safe distance behind. If you do decide to get behind a competitor, then let them know, via auditory cues like breathing or speaking to them, that you are there. Your presence should cause your rival to speed up or make a move on which you can capitalize. A runner with someone behind them, especially a rival, is a runner who may feel pressure to maintain the lead and may eventually drop back. You can control your race from behind them in this way. Deciding to pass them depends on how strong you feel and how much further you have to go. Another mental strategy to practice is the concept of mindfulness. As you are out on the race course, take stock of your rivals. How does their proverbial "system" look? How are they carrying their arms? Are they running effortlessly and efficiently? How is their posture? Are they leaning too far forward? Listen for their breathing. Is it pained and wheezy? Being mindful of your rivals is a good way to understand them. As you run behind them, you can also look for cues that they are starting to fade. Wait a mile or two and compare their form and breathing. Did anything change? If so, they may be vulnerable and ready to be passed.

- **Know when to make your "move."** The stereotypical "race to the finish" always makes for a good story. Seeing rivals duking it out, stride for stride, as they look for every last ounce of energy within a few meters from the finish-line tape is what racing is all about. But just know that if you find yourself in a footrace with a rival, you don't have to wait until the end to make your "move." In fact, a well-timed kick at the start or in the middle of the race may be enough to get past your competition. If you find yourself in a toe-to-toe race then think about not just making that important "move" but when and how to make it. Any "move" usually means a sudden surge of pace. If you have been following the 10K training schedule, then you have done "speed burst" workouts. Making a passing move is one of the reasons for this kind of training. Before you make the move, do a quick "system check" to gauge whether or not your body is prepared. Also, look up and scan the course ahead of you. What does the next 100 to 200 meters look like? Do you have a large hill approaching? If so, you may want to wait for the hill as not only have you done speed burst training, but you have also done hill training, and a good place to make a move on a course is at a challenging point when everyone is suffering equally. Another thing to look for in your course scan is a bottleneck or narrow stretch of course. You want to have a wide berth to make your move. When you do make your move, do it with gusto. Try to pass your rival as if they were standing still. This kind of jolt will give you a mental edge, making them feel as if they have no chance to counter because you are in much better shape than they are. Keep your surge going for at least 20 to 30 seconds, and, if possible, try to get to a point in the course—at a turn, for example—where they lose eye contact with you.

- **Befriend your competitors.** This isn't boxing; it's running. Even though you may show tenacity and aggressiveness out on the roads, it doesn't mean that you hold any kind of personal grudge against your competitors. If you do manage to pass a rival in a race, be sure to find them at the finish and shake their hand. Congratulate them on their own race and thank them for pushing you. The same goes if a rival was able to get the better of you on a particular day. Ask them what their racing plans and training goals are and find out if they live near you. Races are wonderful places to meet future training partners.

Reaching for The "Half"

If you've seriously been bitten by the running "bug" and you've raced both a 5K and a 10K, then you may feel compelled to go even further. A logical next step would be the half-marathon (13.1 miles). However, I caution you to perfect your craft in races under the 10K for at least a year before moving "up" in distance. While doing a half may be a real possibility for you, I believe you will set yourself up for a better racing experience by focusing more on your shorter-distance races for at least a year. You will learn a lot about yourself training for these races that you can capitalize on when you do decide to go for the half marathon. Before you think about the half, try to achieve these milestones first:

- Successfully race a 5K and a 10K without any walk breaks.
- Improve your 5K and 10K personal bests at least three times for each distance.
- Race a trail 5K or 10K.
- Compete in a cross-country race.
- Complete a 60-minute run without any walk breaks.

By no means are these criteria exhaustive, but I just want to caution you a bit. Going too far too soon can lead to injury. Go slow and steady with race-distance progression. This solid foundation will allow you to thrive in the half marathon, and even, someday, the marathon.

The sky truly is the limit, and I don't want you to lose this newfound passion you've found in running, but remember, gradualism is the name of the game. This important, step-by-step, building-block approach is imperative to your long-term success as a runner.

The Best Way to End This Book

Beginning a book about running is the easy part; ending it isn't easy. I have so much that I want to tell you about this wonderful sport. But what I've offered here should provide you the right amount of direction and advice for you to succeed. Do I have more tips and tricks that I'd to impart to you? Absolutely. But there comes a time when you start to learn not from your coach or an author of a book, but from yourself. To that end, I have one final thing I'd like to ask of you. Think back to the first day that you picked up this book. In the first chapter, I taught you about the concept of the equilibrium shift. I asked you to fill out a few questions.

Here They Are

1. The number of minutes you exercise every day: _____
2. The number of days a week that you exercise: _____
3. Describe your eating habits: _____
4. What types of food do you eat most often? _____
5. How often do you snack during the day? _____
6. What kind of snacks do you eat? _____
7. How much water do you drink? _____
8. How much sleep do you get per night? _____
9. Estimate how many hours a day that you are sedentary (watching screens or sitting at your desk): _____
10. How many extra pounds would you like to lose thanks to running? _____

Go ahead and fill these out as the new you.

Now, find your signed contract and the original answers to your questions. Compare your answers.

They don't look the same, do they? These differences reveal one truly impressive accomplishment—you have completed your equilibrium shift.

Be proud.

Take what you've learned· and apply this concept in other facets of your life. Remember that you will always encounter resistant forces when you want to make positive changes.

But wellness is always worth the sacrifice.

CHARTS AND
WORKSHEETS

The Four "Ps" of any Runner

Perseverance
Patience
Passion
Prioritization

Training Maxims

Training Maxim #1	Doing something is better than doing nothing.
Training Maxim #2	Running isn't a recipe.
Training Maxim #3	You will have good training days and you will have bad training days.

Weekly Purpose Table

Purpose Type	Description
Rest and Recover	In this week, you are giving your body a break after a longer period of hard weeks before it. This week will help you ensure you recover your energy and allow your muscles to rest so that you can build in subsequent weeks and minimize the risk of injury.
Base Building	This week is all about building muscular strength and endurance so that you can run longer and faster. Think of it as laying the right, solid foundation that you can build on in subsequent weeks with Hills or Speed Work.
Hills or Speed Work	Typically these are your hardest weeks where you will be running faster and with more intensity in the other two weeks.

Eleven Motivational Tips

1.	Get a loved one to literally push you out the door.
2.	Change up your pace.
3.	Treat yourself.
4.	Set yourself up for success.
5.	Find strength in numbers.
6.	Get pumped.
7.	Establish a routine.
8.	Run different places.
9.	Tell yourself, "One more minute."
10.	Write it out.
11.	Listen to your body and take a zero.